W0114413

Praise for
Restorative Embodiment and Resilience

"This book slowed me down, woke me up, and brought me home. As I read, I was over and over again returned to a restorative state—a deep breath here, a relaxation there—until a newfound sense of rest began to permeate my life. This is the handbook for transmuting fear, grief, and anger into peace, quiet acceptance, love, and open-hearted connection. Ultimately, it's a book about letting all of your feelings come alive in the most restorative and enriching ways imaginable. A gem."

> **AMANDA BLAKE**, Master Somatic Coach, founder of Embright, and author of *Your Body Is Your Brain*

"Deeply informative and a pleasure to read, this book awakens our embodied states of being in everyday life. The author offers skills to transform challenging feelings, dysregulating life habits, and relationships. Slow down, savor these pages, and stay tuned for wonderful case examples and exercises that provide a pathway to deep well-being."

> **TINA STROMSTED**, PhD, LMFT, Jungian psychoanalyst, dance/movement therapist, somatics educator, and director of Soul's Body Center

"Fogel confirms the existence of what he calls *restorative embodied self-awareness*: a deeply relaxing state of being fully present to felt experience that releases the vital capacity humans have to heal our thoughts, emotions, and physical selves. In the process, Fogel explains how feelings such as awe in nature, transcendence, and spiritual connection transform our sense of ourselves and our being in the world. A useful, informative, clear, and compelling treasure of a book!"

> **KIMERER L. LAMOTHE**, PhD, author of *Why We Dance*

"This is an honest book. It brings us back to feeling fully alive in the account of restorative embodied self-awareness (as opposed to dysregulated or modulated embodied self-awareness) that leads us to the present moment of experiencing thoughts, felt sensations, and emotions arising from within our bodies. Excellently selected literature and useful restorative tools make the book a rich source of enlightenment and usability. A must-read for anyone who wants to make the most out of the embodied experience."

SABINE C. KOCH, PhD, director of the Research Institute of Creative Arts Therapies and professor of dance movement therapy at SRH University, Heidelberg, Germany

"Why do we attribute healing to mysterious forces such as placebos without recognizing the role of the embodied self? How is it that in most people the precursors of gut distress lie outside their day-to-day awareness? Fogel speaks to such issues. His book is a definite read for anyone wishing to explore the different attributes of embodied awareness."

DONALD BAKAL, PhD, professor emeritus at the University of Calgary and author of *Minding the Body*

"Whilst there is still a tendency for many living in the modern world to approach life as though mind and body are separate, as Alan rightly states, this is simply wrong—we do not *have* a body, 'we *are* a body.' To truly embody this offers the possibility to transform our conscious experience of ourselves and of the wider world and all our relationships within it. The journey is long, and there is no one path or formula that works for all. At this time of unprecedented change and turmoil on our beautiful Earth, there has never been a more crucial moment to commit to reclaiming our wholeness."

LOUISE LIVINGSTONE, PhD, director of Heart Sense Research Institute, cofounder of the Centre for Myth, Cosmology and the Sacred, and author of *How Can the Thought of the Heart Offer Effective Ways of Engaging with Conflict?*

"Alan Fogel successfully interweaves neurobiological knowledge with research evidence and clinical expertise. A framework is developed to find peace and restoration in the courageous encounter with those aspects of human experience that might, at first, seem unbearable to face. A must-read for beginners and experienced practitioners in embodied experiencing alike."

MANON M. BARTSCH, MA, SRH University, Heidelberg, Germany

"*Restorative Embodiment and Resilience* presents a framework for understanding the interplay of emotional attunement and self-awareness and the critical role of embodied presence for enhancing regulation, embodiment, and health. This book is not about one particular therapeutic approach; rather, it highlights the types of daily interactions with people and nature that can draw us into restorative embodied experience, and the types of therapeutic approaches that can support our capacity to live more deeply in connection with ourselves."

CYNTHIA PRICE, PhD, MA, LMT, research professor at the University of Washington School of Nursing and director of Center for Mindful Body Awareness

"*Restorative Embodiment and Resilience* offers fresh insights to anyone seeking to navigate a course to emotional well-being. Displaying compassion, a breadth of interdisciplinary research, and a wisdom born of personal experience, Fogel identifies and illuminates three states of embodied self-awareness. Fogel also offers the reader the tools needed to access a newly described state of restoration, one in which the work of metabolizing our life's experience can take place. This book is an invaluable resource for anyone seeking to find greater ease within their own being and with the world around them."

PHILIP SHEPHERD, author of *Radical Wholeness*

"Alan Fogel has written a work of extraordinary synthesis and profound depth. His model of *restorative embodied self-awareness* bridges mindfulness, cutting-edge brain science, and deep clinical understanding to create a unique bringing together of so much that is excitingly new in science, alongside ancient wisdom and clinical thinking—all with body awareness at its heart. This book will be a boon for readers interested in gaining an understanding of how embodied awareness can facilitate processes of psychic healing and growth."

GRAHAM MUSIC, PhD, consultant psychotherapist at Tavistock Clinic, London, and author of *Nurturing Children*

"With hours of sitting and staring into computer and phone screens, or getting immersed in virtual reality, the need for embodied presence becomes ever more urgent. And how this embodied presence—and probably any attempt at maintaining resilience in times of uncertainty and trauma—needs to be anchored in our felt sense is solidly presented in this book. Committing to the process of embodiment and the cultivation of presence—be it as a student, client, patient, practitioner, or curious reader—is the real thing."

WOLF E. MEHLING, MD, professor at the University of California, San Francisco, School of Medicine

"Alan's excellent book expresses a deep understanding of embodiment, and I recommend it highly. A profound and also practical work that coaches, therapists, and movement teachers will get a lot from. Take a breath, and dive in!"

MARK WALSH, author of *Embodiment* and founder of The Embodiment Conference

Restorative Embodiment and Resilience

Restorative Embodiment and Resilience

A Guide to Disrupt Habits,
Create Inner Peace,
Deepen Relationships,
and Feel Greater Presence

ALAN FOGEL

Foreword by Stuart G. Shanker, D Phil

North Atlantic Books
Berkeley, California

Copyright © 2021 by Alan Fogel. All rights reserved. No portion of this book, except for brief review, may be reproduced, stored in a retrieval system, or transmitted in any form or by any means—electronic, mechanical, photocopying, recording, or otherwise—without the written permission of the publisher. For information contact North Atlantic Books.

Published by
North Atlantic Books
Berkeley, California

Illustrations by Guy Ruggiero, Pristine Graphics
Cover art ©gettyimages.com/Benjavisa
Cover design by Jennifer Durant
Book design by Happenstance Type-O-Rama

Printed in the United States of America

Restorative Embodiment and Resilience: A Guide to Disrupt Habits, Create Inner Peace, Deepen Relationships, and Feel Greater Presence is sponsored and published by North Atlantic Books, an educational nonprofit based in Berkeley, California, that collaborates with partners to develop cross-cultural perspectives, nurture holistic views of art, science, the humanities, and healing, and seed personal and global transformation by publishing work on the relationship of body, spirit, and nature.

North Atlantic Books' publications are distributed to the US trade and internationally by Penguin Random House Publishers Services. For further information, visit our website at www.northatlanticbooks.com.

MEDICAL DISCLAIMER: The following information is intended for general information purposes only. Individuals should always see their health care provider before administering any suggestions made in this book. Any application of the material set forth in the following pages is at the reader's discretion and is their sole responsibility.

Library of Congress Cataloging-in-Publication Data

Names: Fogel, Alan, author.
Title: Restorative embodiment and resilience : a guide to disrupt habits, create inner peace, deepen relationships, and feel greater presence / Alan Fogel.
Description: Berkeley, California: North Atlantic Books, [2021] | Includes bibliographical references and index.
Identifiers: LCCN 2021001735 (print) | LCCN 2021001736 (ebook) | ISBN 9781623175542 (trade paperback) | ISBN 9781623175559 (ebook)
Subjects: LCSH: Somesthesia. | Self-consciousness (Awareness)
Classification: LCC QP448 .F643 2021 (print) | LCC QP448 (ebook) | DDC 612.8—dc23
LC record available at https://lccn.loc.gov/2021001735
LC ebook record available at https://lccn.loc.gov/2021001736

1 2 3 4 6 7 8 9 KPC 26 25 24 23 22 21

This book includes recycled material and material from well-managed forests. North Atlantic Books is committed to the protection of our environment. We print on recycled paper whenever possible and partner with printers who strive to use environmentally responsible practices.

Contents

Foreword

Alan Fogel has written not just the book that is desperately needed at the present moment in time but a book for the ages. We are not the first society that has become deeply polarized and will certainly not be the last. We are not the first to see neighbors and even families torn apart by conflicting views about the nature of the problems that beset us and how these should be addressed. Not unique in the proliferation of depression and anxiety, loneliness and despair, self-harm and addiction. Not the first that has been subjected to a devastating plague, and not the first to have devastated our environment.

Every age has come up with its own unique way of conceptualizing its societal ills. Maybe the source of the problems lay with capricious gods; or an imbalance in bodily humors; or in the human propensity to sin; or in unconscious drives. Accordingly, maybe the way to restore harmony is by propitiating the gods; bloodletting and cupping; prayer; psychoanalysis.

What makes *Restorative Embodiment and Resilience* such an important turning point is that Fogel provides us with a new way of understanding why so many individuals have become dysregulated—and more important, what we need to do if we are ever to return to a state of harmony at both the personal and the societal level.

The answer is to be found not in entrails or dream analysis but in recent advances in the neuroscience and psychophysiology of embodied self-awareness (ESA). Fogel focuses on the three basic states: *dysregulated, modulated*, and *restorative*. He clarifies what is happening inside our brain and body in each, and what we can do to shift from dysregulated to modulated ESA, with the ultimate goal of restoring restorative ESA in our lives.

He lays out in meticulous detail the biological reasons why restorative ESA is vital, and for that matter, elusive. Ours is a culture that has devised any number of ways to remain in a state of heightened sympathetic arousal, which places a heavy strain on metabolic processes of repair and renewal. The more we overtax our energy system the more dysregulated we become, profoundly affecting what we think and feel. We become anxious and ruminative, our mind caught in endlessly repeating scripts, incapable of constructive and cooperative problem solving.

The hardest part of being dysregulated is simply becoming aware of the fact. We end up doing the very things that keep us dysregulated. This is one of the major reasons why our society has become so polarized. We become increasingly desperate to convince our adversaries that they are destroying the common good. But the more stridently we argue for our position the more polarized we all become: the less able to process what each other is feeling and saying, the less inclined to even try. Our ability to problem-solve is blocked by emotionally charged scripts that impair our ability to listen to each other, or indeed to our own body.

What is most urgently needed when an individual or a society is dysregulated is restoration, not rhetoric. But restorative ESA is not to be confused with some sort of nirvana-like state, where problems simply dissipate. Rather, it is to become fully aware of what we are feeling, physically or emotionally—to become conscious of painful sensations or emotions that we have sought to cope with by avoiding or denying their very existence.

Exposing suppressed and repressed feelings to the full glare of self-awareness has a profoundly detoxifying effect, triggering cellular changes in our hormonal, digestive, and immune systems. But this is not the sort of healing state that can be attained by an act of will. Not by argument, no matter how eloquent. And neither, for that matter, by simply becoming aware of the benefits of restorative ESA.

One of the most powerful messages of the book is that these experiences "come spontaneously and without conceptual thought or focused attention or planning." But for the neural shift that makes this possible, we need to cultivate a state of modulated self-awareness. The first and critical step in this process is to recognize the signs of dysregulation; figure out and reduce the myriad stresses that have landed us in this state; and most important of all, start to build "restorative moments" into our lives.

Each of us has to figure out our own unique pathway to restorative ESA: the experiences that we find truly therapeutic. But one of the central themes in the book is the insight that this process of self-discovery is not something that we can manage on our own. The human brain is so designed that restoration is a function of social engagement: as much at the end of life as at the beginning. We need a secure interbrain presence in order to expose feelings that we have suppressed or repressed precisely because we find them so threatening.

By no means is this argument meant to suggest that, only now, with the development of neuro-imaging technologies, are we able to identify the three states of ESA. But with understanding of the relationship between prefrontal systems and psychological states or emotions comes a deeper insight into—a reframing—of some of the pivotal moments of restorative ESA in the history of our civilization. Beginning with the Revelation that occurred at Sinai: a time when a "burdensome, bothersome, and quarrelsome" people (Deut. 1:12) managed to listen to themselves and to each other and so speak with one voice (Deut. 24:7).

More than anything, this is a book that inspires the profound sense of hope that such a momentous event can occur again. There is never a moment when we can't begin to restore restoration. When we can't come a step closer to understanding ourselves and bettering the human condition. But we can't begin to resolve a problem until we understand the nature of that problem. And that, ultimately, is the reason why *Restorative Embodiment and Resilience* is such a momentous book. It brings us a critical step closer to understanding ourselves and bettering the human condition.

Stuart G. Shanker, D Phil (Oxon)

Distinguished Research Professor Emeritus
of Philosophy and Psychology, York University
Founder and CEO, The MEHRIT Centre
Founder and Visionary, Self-Reg Global
Author, Reframed: Self-Reg for a Just Society
January 2021

Preface

This is a book about restorative embodied self-awareness (ESA), a state of being that involves a sense of peace, safety, connection, oneness, and being completely in the present moment. When we are in a state of restorative ESA, there is no past or future. There is only now. There is complete immersion in the sea of felt experience. There are no explanatory or narrative thoughts in this state, only evocative words or images that resonate with the felt experience, that expand it and give it a sense of "truth."

Restorative ESA is not necessarily a state of happiness, although the felt experience of happiness may be part of it. We can also be fully present with pain, grief, anger, shame, or memories of trauma and horror in ways that make them restorative. This complete presence with whatever we are feeling has the power to transform those feelings, to detoxify them, and to alter the cellular physiology of the body in ways that promote whole-body restoration and recovery.

When we genuinely and wholly embrace our feelings of shame, or of not being enough, for example, these felt experiences have the opportunity to become metabolized through all the functional systems of the body. This means that they are less likely to cause illness or despair, less likely to paralyze us, less likely to keep us from becoming who we really are, our "true self" that has been hidden behind or underneath all of the loss and pain that are part of the human condition.

Restorative states cannot be "explained" or even described in narrative language. Language can only point toward those states because their "content" is nonlinguistic. They are composed of felt experiences that can only be appreciated in the present moment of feeling them. So, writing a book about these states is a fraught endeavor.

One approach to writing taken here is by using contrast. We can use language to describe the other states of embodied self-awareness, of which there are two: *dysregulated* and *modulated*. Much of this book, except for the last chapter, which is devoted entirely to restorative ESA, is about making these contrasts and using examples of what it might feel like to be in dysregulated, modulated, or restorative ESA. These contrasts can help you better understand the state in which you may be living at any moment in time.

Another approach is by explaining the anatomy and physiology that supports each of these three states of ESA. Awareness, including self-awareness, would not be possible without a particular kind of nervous system. When we talk about awareness of things outside the self, we mean the part of the nervous system and sense organs that make up the five senses. This book is about self-awareness: the ways in which we perceive, feel, and understand the inner condition of our body.

Self-awareness comes from the brain, the spinal cord, and the peripheral nervous system (which extends throughout the body to transfer information about body feelings and actions to and from the brain). If these anatomical discourses are not to your liking, feel free to skip over them. They are primarily contained in the first two chapters.

If we just said that there is a dedicated part of the nervous system for embodied self-awareness, the anatomy is simply a stand-in for what we already know and experience. We don't need to know the anatomy of the vocal organs and muscles of speech articulation, or about the language centers of the brain, in order to speak and listen. We don't need to know how our car works in order to drive it. Somebody else, the doctor or the auto mechanic, needs to know these things but maybe not us.

If you are a doctor or therapist or embodied educator, then you might find this information helpful to your practice. It will give you a better understanding of how people respond to embodied interventions and treatments and suggest ways to work with particular states of ESA.

Another reason to include this anatomical information is that each of the states has a unique impact on the health of all our body systems, even the ones that have nothing to do with self-awareness. You might want to know the physiology of why and how staying in prolonged states of dysregulated ESA can lead to a host of serious and even life-threatening illnesses.

This knowledge about the harmful effects of dysregulation is useful, for sure, and it is also very well-known. There are literally thousands of books and research studies about how unresolved trauma and stress, prolonged anxiety and depression, or unchecked aggression can make you sick, very sick. You can find a review of some of these findings in this book and references to this larger body of work that you can follow up if you desire.

More central to the theme of this book, however, is: What makes restorative ESA restorative? What is the physiology that allows states of peace and relaxation to actually heal trauma, physical illnesses, and many forms of mental malaise? How does "mere" self-awareness engender cellular changes in the cardiovascular, respiratory, hormonal, immune, sexual and reproductive, and digestive systems of the body that lead to observable reductions in pain and suffering? What is it about allowing ourselves direct access to felt experience that contributes to health and well-being, even if that felt experience is challenging, difficult, or painful?

Even if you skip over these anatomical details, you will still get a lot from reading this book. It will give you some concrete, actionable tools to break out of unproductive habits in order to improve your well-being, health, relationships, and peace within yourself.

A third approach to writing about restorative ESA, and the other two states, is by giving examples from everyday life. There are many quotes from ordinary individuals who describe in their own words the felt experience of being in different states. Also included are quotes from books and research studies that were chosen to be illustrative of restoration, modulation, and dysregulation. These quotes may help you identify similar feelings within yourself.

Here is a brief outline of each chapter. There is no need to read linearly from start to finish. Begin with whatever calls your attention. Let that lead you back to pick up any information that might enhance your grasp of what you chose as a starting point. If you get stuck on something, skip to something else. Slow down as needed. Reread as needed. See what touches you and what annoys you. It's now in your hands.

Chapter 1: Embodied Self-Awareness: Staying in Touch—and Losing Touch—with Ourselves and Others

This chapter presents an overview of the theme of embodied self-awareness, the present-moment experiencing of the thoughts, felt sensations, and emotions that arise from within our bodies. Felt sensations can be classified into four categories: interoception, proprioception, autonomic nervous system feelings, and emotional feelings. This chapter gives examples of some of these felt experiences and explains why they are essential to our survival and well-being. Comparisons are made between thinking about ourselves vs. feeling ourselves. The neurophysiology of thinking in the default-mode and task-positive cognitive networks will be described. This chapter also introduces the idea that felt experience is compromised or diminished by thinking and that it is distorted and dysregulated by stress and trauma.

Chapter 2: Three States of Embodied Self-Awareness and Four Forms of Felt Experience

This chapter briefly introduces the three different ways in which we can experience our ESA: restorative, modulated, and dysregulated. These differences in embodied experience come from our life histories, including traumatic ones, that moved us to either embrace (restorative ESA), learn to manage (modulated ESA), or avoid (dysregulated ESA) our felt experiences including emotions and body sensations. The neurophysiology and self-awareness of the four types of felt experience are explained in detail.

Chapter 3: Three States of Embodied Self-Awareness: Felt Experience, Thinking, and Autonomic Nervous System Activation

Each of the three different states of ESA has a different type of thought process, a different type of felt experience, and a different signature of activity in the autonomic nervous system (ANS). This chapter answers such questions as: What is felt experience and how does that relate to each state of ESA? What kinds of thought processes enhance or get in the way of felt experience? What is the ANS, and why is it important to our understanding of the three states of ESA?

Chapter 4: The Felt Experience of Maintaining or Changing States of Embodied Self-Awareness

Most of us, most of the time, are in either modulated or dysregulated ESA. Transforming these states into a state of restorative ESA takes practice and guidance. This chapter presents the idea that we can learn to feel when we shift or change from one state of ESA to another. The ability to shift out of dysregulated states is essential for self-care and self-repair. Everyday examples of the three states and how we can shift between them provide readers with some tools to deepen their own embodied awareness.

Chapter 5: Out of the Ordinary: Pain, Eating, and Breathing during the Three States of Embodied Self-Awareness

In this chapter there are examples of how some of our everyday body sensations may feel in each of the three states of ESA, along with a discussion of how we shift between those states. The felt experiences reviewed in this chapter are chosen because they are common, basic, and ordinary types of body experience: the interoception of pain, the interoception and proprioception related to eating and body shape/size/appearance, and the interoceptive and autonomic felt experiences of breathing.

Chapter 6: How Our State of Embodied Self-Awareness Affects Emotional Experiences

In this chapter we explore many different types of emotional experiences, including anger/rage, fear/anxiety, enjoyment/pleasure, sadness/grief, and shame/embarrassment. Although a lot has been written about emotion, and although emotion is something we experience every day, this chapter provides a new perspective that has never been explored: that the "same" emotion, such as fear, is experienced differently in each of the three states of ESA. Allowing ourselves to completely embrace a feeling of fear can be restorative if we can stop avoiding the feeling. This gives us the possibility to become empowered by it. Pleasure, to take another example, can be destructively dysregulated when addictions, violence, and hatred become self-centered, criminal, and/or appalling sources of satisfaction for the perpetrator.

Chapter 7: Experiences of Restorative Embodied Self-Awareness: In Their Own Words

Unlike the previous chapters in which we looked at the differences between dysregulated, modulated, and restorative ESA, this final chapter focuses primarily on restorative ESA. While previous chapters provided some examples of individuals' descriptions of their different states of ESA, this chapter contains personal descriptions of what it feels like to be in restorative ESA. The writings quoted for this chapter did not specifically mention the word *restoration* but rather were chosen because they illustrate the basic principles of restorative ESA as described in chapter 3: there is a felt parasympathetic state of rest; the feelings come spontaneously and without conceptual thought or focused attention or planning; and we are able to slow down, let go, surrender to being fully in the moment, to allow our attention to be broad and free-floating—in other words, without "doing," effort, or deliberate control.

This book is dedicated to everyone who has had the courage, or seeks to have the courage, to move out of dysregulation and embark on the unknowable path that leads to the feelings of peace, relaxation, wholeness, and personal integrity that come with restoration.

The journey is long, filled with temptations to disembark, goes backward, gets worse before it gets better, and there is no one path, no formula that works for everyone, no highways or express transports.

May you encounter the guidance, love, safety, supports, and resources that find you when you get lost and that remind you that there is hope even when all you see is despair.

Embodied
Self-Awareness

Staying in Touch—and Losing Touch—with Ourselves and Others

Embodied self-awareness (ESA) refers to the ways in which we pay attention to what is happening inside of our own body. ESA has two basic forms. We can be aware of the felt experiences from within the body, or we can be aware of our thoughts about ourselves. We can feel ourselves, or we can think about ourselves, but usually not both at the same time. These two forms of self-awareness arise from completely different networks in the nervous system.

These separate networks have unique connections between the brain and the parts of the nervous system that extend through the body, and they have direct effects on virtually all body functions, each in its own way. This means that being aware of our thoughts and feelings has the potential to improve our mental and physical health and well-being, our ability to move and accomplish tasks in our lives, and our relationships to other people. On the other hand, a lack of awareness about what we think or feel about ourselves—either because of deliberate avoidance or because of stressful or traumatic conditions that keep our attention focused outside of ourselves— can impair other body functions.

The concept of embodied self-awareness encompasses the whole of what people talk about when they use the words *mind* and *body*. *Mind* often means our thoughts and mental images. *Mind* can also refer to the brain or what goes on "in the head" as opposed to in the body. This kind of talk can be confusing because the head and the brain are actually part of the body. The head and brain are attached at the neck by nerves, bones, muscles, and fascia that link the head and its functional and sensory organs with the other parts of the body.

The brain in the head is linked to the rest of the body via the nervous system, hormones, and blood that travel throughout the whole body. The brain, indeed, is in the head, and those nerve cells connect into the brain stem and spinal cord to form links to the peripheral nervous system in all the other parts of the body that are not the head (see Figure 1.1). Anything that we can feel in our bodies, any movements that we make, any emotional expressions, any actions in the body depend on the two-way communication between the brain and peripheral nervous systems and the blood and hormones that circulate between the brain and the rest of the body.

If nerves are severed in any part of the body, we can't feel that part or move it anymore. On the other hand, if the parts of the brain that receive signals from a specific part of the peripheral nervous system are damaged—such as from a stroke or head injury—we lose feeling and movement in those linked peripheral locations in the body. So even at a basic physiological level, the so-called mind and so-called body are one and the same. In this book, we'll use the word *embodied* as a way to include the head and the brain and the thoughts that seem to be coming from our head along with all our other tissues and cells, like those in the skin and muscles and bones and organ systems.

The brain, in addition to neurally linking to the rest of the body, controls secretions of substances called *hormones* into the blood. Hormones regulate many different types of body functions like digestion, urination, body temperature, metabolism, and reproductive and sexual function. In fact, the

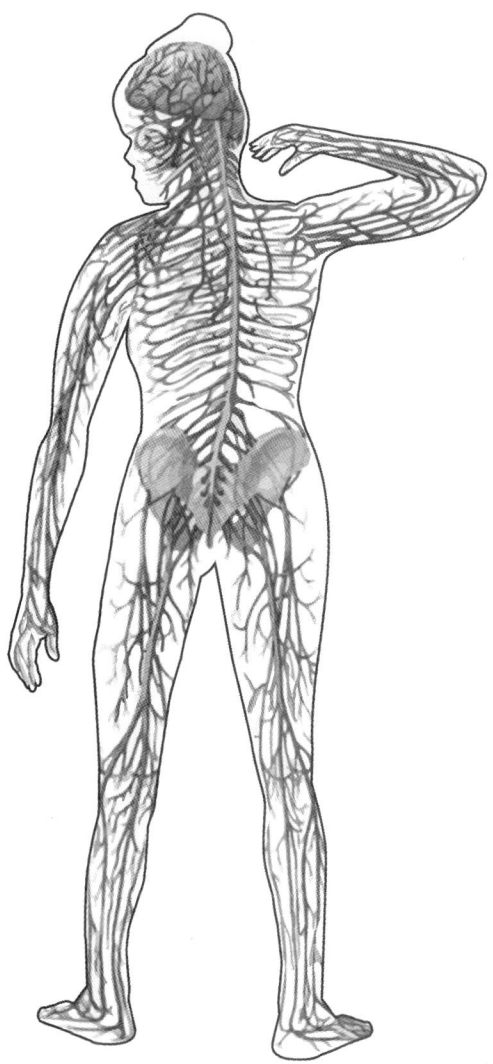

FIGURE 1.1: *The nervous system extends throughout the whole body.*

bloodstream, because of its microscopic capillaries, touches all the cells of the body. The peripheral nervous system, on the other hand, does not reach all the cells of the body. Peripheral nerve endings (called *receptors*) are connected to groups of cells rather than to individual cells.

This brain-to-blood linkage begins at the base of the brain in a region called the *hypothalamus*. The hypothalamus is connected into brain networks above it that sense whether we need to prepare for some type of activity (like responding to a danger, exercise, work, or a sexual encounter) or to slow down and rest. Underneath the hypothalamus is the pituitary gland. These two organs work together to create the many different kinds of hormones that are secreted into the blood (Figure 1.2). The hypothalamus also has neural connections (specifically, through the autonomic nervous system, as explained in detail throughout chapters 2 and 3) to the rest of the body via the brain stem and peripheral nerves, making it an essential brain-to-body control center.

To take one example, the hormone ACTH is secreted from the pituitary gland when other parts of the brain sense—because of both blood chemistry and peripheral nerves' signals from the body coming back to the brain—that the body needs metabolic energy to complete a task, exercise, or respond to a threat or challenge. ACTH cells in the blood eventually reach the adrenal glands, located on top of the kidneys in the mid-lower back region. The adrenals convert ACTH into another hormone, cortisol, a blood sugar that boosts energy and is also a neurotransmitter.

This means that when the cortisol-laden blood returns to the brain, it creates a feedback loop to assist the body in increasing or decreasing the amount of cortisol needed. The hypothalamus and pituitary also create hormones for interpersonal warmth and closeness (oxytocin). They produce hormones for sexual activity (penile and clitoral erections and sexual arousal, genital lubrication, and orgasm) and reproduction (sperm and ova release in the gonadal glandular system and milk release in the lactating glands of the breasts). These brain centers also create the hormonal precursors to release metabolic resources in the thyroid glands and in other glandular systems for temperature regulation and cellular growth.

Like cortisol, all the hormones that circulate around the body in the bloodstream also perfuse brain cells and act as neurotransmitters that affect brain function. When our sexual encounter has ended, for example, the reduction of sex hormones that enter the central nervous system signals the hypothalamus to slow or stop the production of those hormones. Similarly, when we finish our exercise session or stop working, the body-to-brain connection turns off or slows down the production of ACTH and cortisol.

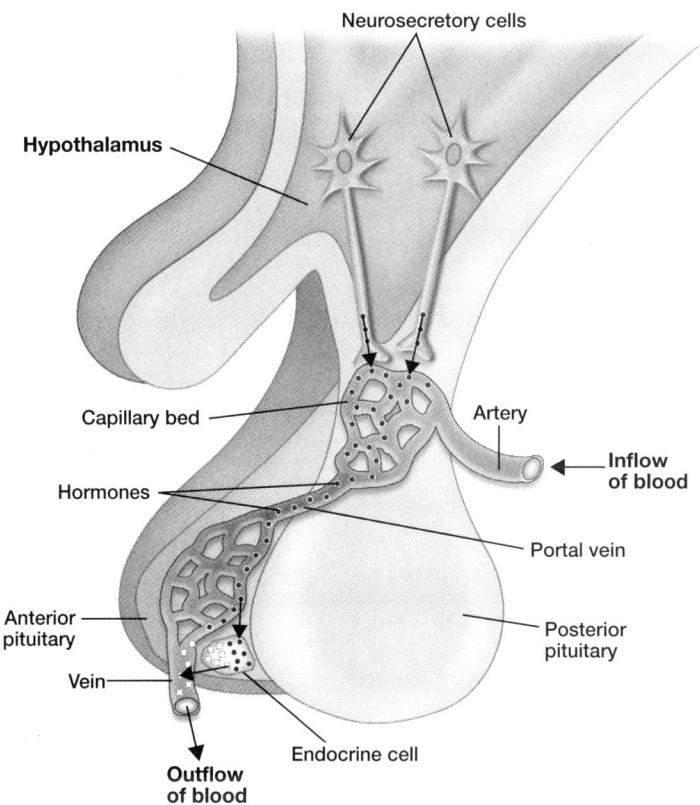

Neurosecretory cells

Hypothalamus

Capillary bed

Artery

Inflow
of blood

Hormones

Portal vein

Anterior
pituitary

Posterior
pituitary

Vein

Outflow
of blood

Endocrine cell

FIGURE 1.2: *The hypothalamus and pituitary respond to information from the brain to create a variety of hormones that are secreted into the bloodstream.*

Coming back to the theme of the unity of "mind" and "body," there are many more connections between the head and the rest of the body than between the brain and body via the nervous system and bloodstream. The nostril passages and mouth are connected to the trachea and lungs. The mouth connects via the throat and esophagus to the entire digestive system and all of its organs (like the stomach, intestines, liver, pancreas, and gallbladder), as well as to the kidneys, bladder, and urinary tract. Vocalizations from the mouth are created in the diaphragm, chest, and throat. The tongue is a muscle that connects into the muscles of the neck, which in turn connect to other muscles that attach to bones in the chest and shoulders. The eyes and ears, via the entire nervous and neuromuscular systems, affect head turning and body movements toward or away from sights and sounds.

All these head-to-body connections make it difficult to defend the not-very-useful distinction between mind and body. Using the concept of embodied self-awareness better represents the idea that both our thoughts and our feelings are brought into awareness via multicellular pathways that extend throughout the whole body.

By some (devious?) route in the evolution of our species, a form of consciousness was created in which thinking seems as if it comes from someplace inside the head. But the fact is that all our thoughts are founded upon an embodied experience, created within the entire network of the cells, tissues, and structures of a living human body. And conversely, a muscle pain, for example, seems as if it is coming from a particular part of the body (the arm, or leg, or fingers, or wherever). That pain awareness, however, is similarly created by a distributed network of cells in the peripheral nervous system that link to brain centers for bringing the pain into conscious awareness (along with the information that the pain seems "located" at the periphery).

Our conscious experience of ourselves, therefore, feeds into the apparent division of mind and body. As we've just seen, however, we are misled by our experience. You could say that the mind has a body and the body has a mind, but that is just perpetuating the useless dichotomy of the mind-body metaphor. Let's just forget that whole (huge, centuries-old) chunk of cultural and philosophical meandering because it doesn't serve us anymore. It's just plain wrong!

Embodied does not mean we *have* a body: it means that we *are* a body. It means that there is no other way of being human except through our fundamental embodiment.[1] The idea of body ownership (I *have* a body) is a curious metaphor that goes along with the body-mind metaphor, both of which developed in Western industrialized cultures. Our Western notion of ownership, and the fact that we can own many physical possessions, makes it seem natural to talk about the body as thing that we have or something that we own.

In the societal domain of human rights, this metaphor is an important ally for political movements such as women's rights and racial-equality activism. For a woman, or a man, or a transgender or nonbinary person, or a

Black person, or Latinx or Asian person, it seems essential to say clearly that all individuals have personal rights to their own bodies that cannot be taken away by laws, patriarchal restrictions, hatred, endemic violence, or discrimination. In these discourses, it seems that body ownership language has an important place to defend one's personal integrity as a human being.

In human rights discussions, however, people are talking not just about the body as a thing to which we own the rights but about our right to our own personal thoughts and feelings, to our unique human identity and value regardless of external appearance, gender orientation, or skin color. At a deeper level, perhaps the discourse is about the right to our unique individual way of being embodied. Still, given the sociocultural framework that assumes a distinction between mind and body, it makes some sense to frame these discussions in a language that is commonly understood.

Generally speaking, however, the mind-body distinction and the sense that I have a body rather than that I am a body puts the so-called body at a distance from the so-called mind. Some of this kind of thinking comes out of centuries of Western cultural, religious, and philosophical distinctions between thoughts being considered as ethereal and non-corporeal and completely different from the actual flesh, pulsations, and sinews of the body.[2] Again, all this discourse is fundamentally wrong, but that's our cultural inheritance from which we must begin if we are to make effective changes.

In spite of the gains achieved in the rights of women, LGBTQ individuals, and people of color, there still persists an endemic cultural bias that the body—and therefore the person living in that body—is a thing. The pervasiveness of how we look at bodies, and especially our gaze at girls' and women's bodies, perpetuates "learning to experience the body as a thing outside the self, something a woman *has* rather than something she *is*," as author Carolyn Knapp put it.[3] This objectifying gaze includes not only men looking at women but women looking at each other and at themselves (see the section on shame, p. 200).

The objectification of the body leads to a perversion of the idea of embodiment promoted in this book—that is, to a favoring of external cues and evaluations over our own felt experience. While predominant in the Western world, this is not the case in all cultures.

West Africans, for example, test higher on measures of interoceptive awareness compared to Europeans and North Americans, most likely because they have a cultural worldview that emphasizes the holistic connection between the head and the heart. People from East Asian cultures are similarly better than Westerners in assessing their interoceptive awareness. This is most likely based upon centuries of traditional Asian medical and health practices that respect the shared contribution of body states and mental states.[4]

Yes, we inhabitants of Western culture are too busy, too focused, too preoccupied, too much in our heads to stop, slow down, and feel ourselves. But the effects of cultural dichotomies like mind vs. body—built into everyday language—are an unseen, pervasive, and perverse influence in keeping us away from feeling ourselves.

People with migraines, to take one example, may refer to the headache as "it." "Why is *it* happening now?" Accepting the migraines as part of one's whole self and learning via felt experience to pay attention to the muscle tension in the neck and shoulders that precedes the onset of an attack, on the other hand, can lead to reduction of pain and stress. This also changes how people think about their headaches. Migraine-savvy individuals do not have migraines: they are migraine people.[5]

In the case of pregnancy, to take another example, the language is more favorable to the sense of embodiment used here. People say "I am pregnant" rather than "I have a pregnancy." That changes, however, when it comes to giving birth. Researchers compared a group of women during childbirth who were instructed to just feel the sensations of each contraction as it came and went with a group who were given methods to distract themselves from the sensations. The latter group was being asked, essentially, to separate the mind from the body. The women who were asked to attend to the sensations using the felt-experience part of their ESA had less self-reported pain than the women in the distraction group.[6]

You might think that if you pay direct and undivided attention to a pain or discomfort, it would make it worse. The miracle of ESA is that fully embracing our felt experience changes the experience: the pain begins to feel less intense when we actually feel it and accept that it is a part of our embodiment in the present moment. Feeling ourselves in this way can also change the thoughts about that experience. Are you "in labor" or are you "laboring"?

Which of these cultural frameworks best fits you? Are you more likely to say that you *have* a body? Or do you tell yourself that "I *am* my body"? Are you more likely to say "I have a virus" or "I am sick and contagious"? Or what about these statements? "My body has gained a lot of weight recently" vs. "I am getting fat." Or "I have diabetes" vs. "I am a diabetic who needs a special diet and regular injections. It's just part of who I am."

This book makes the point that embracing and accepting what is actually happening in the whole body can often lead to relief and sometimes profound change that contributes to healing. Denying those experiences, or pretending that they are not important, or acting like the mind is safe and sound even though the body is sick, is pretty much a guarantee that the symptoms will get worse. If you wish to find and cultivate your ESA, this book will help you do that with concrete methods and suggestions along with conceptual tools to help the thinking part of yourself understand why your feeling part is essential for well-being.

Embodied Thinking and Embodied Feeling

Embodied self-awareness is *both how we feel and experience ourselves and how we think about ourselves*. ESA also means that *our only access* to the experience of our whole body system is via these two forms of awareness. There is no other way to be embodied. There is no other way to be human.

Feeling and thinking can take many different forms, from the sublime to the ordinary, from love to hate, from passion to detachment. Understanding these different forms of ESA—their content and origins—and the many ways to monitor and regulate our ESA is the subject of this book.

Feeling and thinking, because they arise in different neural networks and have different pathways around the body, are for the most part mutually exclusive. We can't do both at the same time.[7] Whenever thoughts come into our awareness—even thoughts about our felt experience, such as "I wonder what caused this pain" or "I just need to slow down and focus on what I am feeling"—we immediately go off-line from our felt experience.*

To rephrase the earlier statement—that thinking and feeling can't happen at the same time—almost any kind of *thinking is a symptom of an impairment in the ability to sense our felt experience.* Table 1.1 gives a summary of the differences between thinking about ourselves and feeling ourselves.

TABLE 1.1: *Differences between the thinking and feeling components of embodied self-awareness*[†]

THINKING ABOUT OURSELVES	FEELING OURSELVES
The self trying **to explain, understand, and interpret** itself, trying to make sense of things	The self **experiencing** itself, not trying to figure out anything, simply being immersed in feeling
Based in linguistic forms of thought, inner speech, and speech with others. Can also include auditory, tactile, olfactory, and visual images and memories.	Based in interoceptive, proprioceptive, autonomic, and emotional feelings
Rational, logical, explanatory, abstract thought that **transcends the present moment**	Spontaneous, concrete, **lived in the present moment**
Experienced as facts, details, narrative, information, story, insight, ideas, interpretations, self-assessments	Experienced as temperature, pressure, movement, shape, pain, breath, energy level, mood, emotions
Attention is focused, directed, and oriented toward reaching a solution or goal	**Attention is diffuse and free-floating**, not bound by control or effort
GIFT: Can take us anywhere in time and gives us **vision and perspective**	GIFT: Takes us **right here** in time and gives us **aliveness and relief**

---

* I realize this statement is taking a rather extreme position. Some people I have talked to claim that they can do both at the same time. I have not had this experience, and the neural architecture doesn't support this claim. If you feel you can do this, however, then I recommend slowing yourself down and really experimenting with seeing what you can feel when you are thinking. When I am feeling anything in my body, my sense is that the thoughts I was just previously having are somehow still "there" but transparent, faded into a background as residual images, and are no longer thoughts that I can "work on" or that lead anywhere.

† I am grateful to Amanda Blake for allowing me to borrow some of her wording to construct this table. See Amanda Blake, *Your Body Is Your Brain* (Trokay Press, 2018).

Another shared Western cultural practice is that we learn, through formal systems of education, to think and that we are predisposed to think almost all the time. Since we are entirely familiar and practiced in thinking, let's review what it means to feel something coming from inside the body. These self-feelings, or felt experiences, of ESA are composed of *interoceptive, proprioceptive, autonomic*, and *emotional* feelings. These components of felt experience will be covered in more detail in the next chapter, along with a discussion of where they arise in the nervous system. For now, Table 1.2 gives a brief overview.

TABLE 1.2: *Felt experiences that arise from within our bodies*

TYPE OF FELT EXPERIENCE	EXAMPLES OF FEELINGS
Interoception	Pain/ease, warm/cold, illness/health, itchy, nauseous, dizzy, hungry, tingling and chills, strong/shaky, achy, jumpy, bloated, weak, suffocating, numb, tense, flushed, congested, confused, trembling
Proprioception	Balance and equilibrium, feeling the coordination (or lack of coordination) between the arms and legs and trunk of our body in motion, sensing our shape and size (fat, thin, muscular, or sinewy), and sensing our location, distance, and boundaries relative to objects and other people
Autonomic Nervous System	Heartbeat, breathing or breathless, arousal or fatigue, stress or relaxation, energized or tired, sweaty, throbbing, reproductive, sexual and erotic feelings, urinary and digestive feelings
Emotion	Happy, sad, angry, ashamed, afraid, proud, disgusted, excited

Curiously, interoception can also involve feelings about thoughts.[8] There is the feeling when we know something but can't quite recall it at the moment, a "tip of the tongue" feeling. Then there is the feeling that something we hear or see feels familiar, like we have been exposed previously but again can't quite bring the prior situation into memory. A third feeling about thinking is the sense that we are getting close to solving a problem, the sense of coming to a conclusion, or a sense of completion. Finally, there is the sense of boredom, of having heard these thoughts or participated in these conversations, and continued exposure to these thoughts feels tedious or tiring.

Experiential Exercise: Thinking vs. Felt Experience

All the feelings listed in Table 1.2 are familiar. Everyone has felt them at some time but most likely for brief periods. It is so easy to think that we are living fully in the present moment with our felt experience, yet the fact is that we are thinking and not really feeling.

You can experience this attraction to thinking by taking a few minutes right now. First, think about how you feel and have been feeling today and the past few days. You'll find it is fairly easy to generate a sizable list of self-descriptions that are likely to be fairly accurate. You probably will find it challenging to stop thinking so much, but let's try and see what happens.

Instead of trying to *think* about yourself, sit or lie down in a comfortable place, and remove any distractions that might disturb you. This works best if you are in a quiet place.[9] Close your eyes. See if you can slow your thoughts long enough to feel something concrete right in the present moment. It doesn't really matter what you feel, so long as it captures your attention long enough for you to feel it. It could be the hardness or softness of the surface on which you are lying or sitting, the texture of your clothing against your skin, an ache or pain, an itch, your heartbeat, or an emotion that wants to surface.

The initial training in many embodied awareness practices such as mindfulness meditation begins with *focusing* on some concrete feeling, like your breath going in and out or your feet on the floor. Research done at various universities and medical centers in Norway shows that focused attention is not very helpful for accessing felt experience, which needs a more *free-floating or diffuse* kind of attention to the body.[10] Focusing attention will activate an effort to concentrate and control, and it most typically leads into some kind of thinking about whether or not we are doing it right or getting where we think we are supposed to be going with this experiential exercise.

Instead, see if you can allow your attention to yourself to wander about your body. Let the wandering be without any deliberate effort to take a particular route through your body. Body scan meditations, for example, use focused attention, usually starting at the head and working the attention gradually down to the feet, or vice versa. That's not what we want to do here. See if you can resist having a plan or purpose and just let your attention go wherever it finds something to feel, wherever your curiosity takes you.

Maybe there is a feeling of tightness or achiness in your chest. Notice that, and then broaden your attention to see if any other places feel tight like in your face or your belly. Again, you are sensing and feeling without any plan—you are following where your attention "wants" to go. See if there are any emotional feelings such as fear or worry or irritation that go with the tightness, or ache, or pain, or expansiveness, or whatever you feel.

See what thoughts come to you about any of these feelings, and just let them float around in your awareness as you keep coming back to your felt experiences. See if it is possible to do this without any deliberate effort to make the feeling get better, to change it, or to try to understand it. If you feel this urge to fix or change or explain your feeling, just notice that, and let the urge be merely another feeling that is coming up for you. It is not necessary to act on that urge.

Each time you come back to your felt experience, it may "land" in a different part of your body, so just practice letting yourself go wherever that takes you. At some point, if you give yourself enough time, as you are letting your attention wander through the sensations coming from your body, there is likely going to be one or a few sensations or emotions that begin to stand out, that capture your attention and hold it in one place for a least a few minutes. Once again, this attentional capture is not deliberate, not focused. It is someplace you arrive but not because you followed a specific route or plan.

Letting your attention drift around and then get drawn or pulled into a particular feeling endows that feeling with a personal intrinsic motivation to explore it. You don't have to try to focus on it because you are just allowing the feeling to "call" you to it.

How is this calling different from focusing? Being "called" by a felt experience is similar to when you might be busy with something and a friend, child, or partner calls out to you and asks for your attention to something that they need to share with you. If you choose to drop your focus on your goals, plans, and expectations, you can be more open to the other person. You can just listen and take in the other person, what they say to you, and the feelings they express.

A lot of people have trouble just dropping their focus and really listening to themselves or to another person who calls them. If this happens to you, simply notice the pull of the focus, the wanting to not let go of whatever it was that you were working on. See if you can let that be just another feeling to which there is no attachment: it can float by as you let yourself be called by a different feeling or another person.

In this experiential exercise, you are approaching your own body with a similar kind of openness that you might offer to another person, a similar dropping of your plans and expectations, a similar "showing up" in the present moment. You are "listening" to your own body "speaking" to you in its own way, and not because you are supposed to be doing something in particular or trying to control the outcome.

Often this felt experience that captures your attention will get more intense and alive, and you will feel totally one with the experience. And at some point this feeling will begin to fade or soften, and you'll eventually return to your thoughts. But see if you notice any change in yourself after staying with the feeling, like a deeper breath or a sense of relief. Feelings of relief and relaxation are some of the physiological signals indicating that you have allowed yourself to be fully in the present moment with a felt experience.

Felt Experience vs. Task-Oriented Thinking

In the next chapter, we will look in more detail at the neural networks for felt experience. In this chapter, we'll cover two different networks for thinking: the task-positive network and the default-mode network.

As we saw in the experiential exercise, methods designed to enhance body awareness using focused attention are less likely to inspire being fully present with felt experience in a way that leads to a sense of relaxation. This is because any kind of focused attention to a task, even if that task is to pay attention to our body sensations, is going to take some mental effort or concentration. The brain network called the *task-positive network* (TPN) specializes in focusing, problem solving, explaining, guiding, and getting things done. We need this powerful ability to focus in order to work and live and survive.[11]

The main brain regions of the TPN (Figure 1.3) are the dorsolateral prefrontal cortex, the insula, the sensorimotor cortex, and the anterior cingulate cortex. In brain anatomy, the word *cortex* refers to the outer layer of the brain that surrounds a deeper core center of the brain. Generally, thinking is happening in the cortex while felt experience is generated in the core section of the brain.

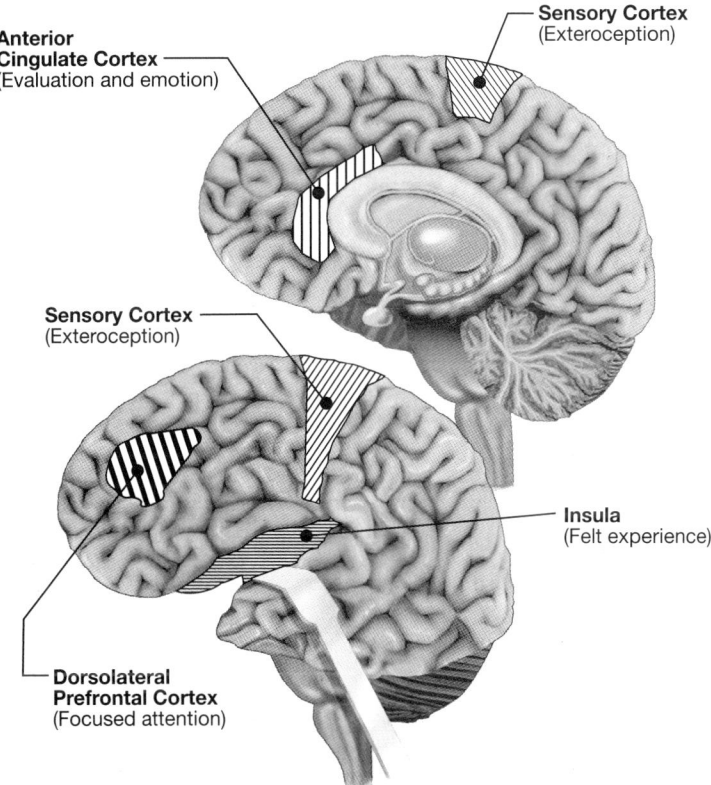

FIGURE 1.3: *The thinking brain: the task-positive network.*

The prefrontal cortex is the part of the brain that is located in the front of the head, above the eyes. The dorso (toward the top of the head) lateral (on the side of the head) prefrontal cortex is the main region that is responsible for focused attention. Internal information arises from a brain network that is connected to the insula that gives us interoception, proprioception, and autonomic feelings. A part of this network is the anterior cingulate cortex, which creates emotional feelings about all the other felt experiences (see Table 1.2 and chapter 2, Figure 2.5, p. 68). External information arises in the sensorimotor cortex from the five senses (also called *exteroception*, compared to interoception) of vision, hearing, smell, taste, and touch.

For the task-positive network, interoception and exteroception are not "allowed" to form lasting felt experiences. Rather, these sensations and feelings are distilled or reduced into the sound bites of thought. The TPN does not dwell on felt experiences nor on taking in a beautiful sunset or listening to music and being moved by it. Instead, the TPN creates words for these feelings, words that lead to productive action, coherent narratives in speech and thought, explanations, judgments, interpretations, and logical reasoning.

It is as if the dorsolateral prefrontal cortex distills and organizes all these senses into "just the facts." "Yup," our TPN might think, "the sun is setting. That's nice. I like the colors. Hey, I'm getting hungry so it must be dinnertime." Or, the interoception of hunger is translated by the TPN into a thought like "What's for dinner?" The TPN pushes us onward, past "mere" feeling or sensation and into action-and-solution mode.

TPN thoughts, as a rule, are linguistic. Sentences scroll out of the auditory cortex and make "sounds" in our heads. The brain areas of the TPN are also linked, therefore, to other areas in the cortex related to speech and language (see Figure 1.4). Broca's area in the lateral posterior (outer layer, toward the back) frontal lobe is linked to the sensory and motor cortices for the production of speech sounds. Wernicke's area, adjacent to the auditory cortex in the temporal lobe (located on the side of the head above the ears), helps with the processing and understanding of speech (our own inner speech thoughts, what we say out loud to others, and the language we hear spoken by others).

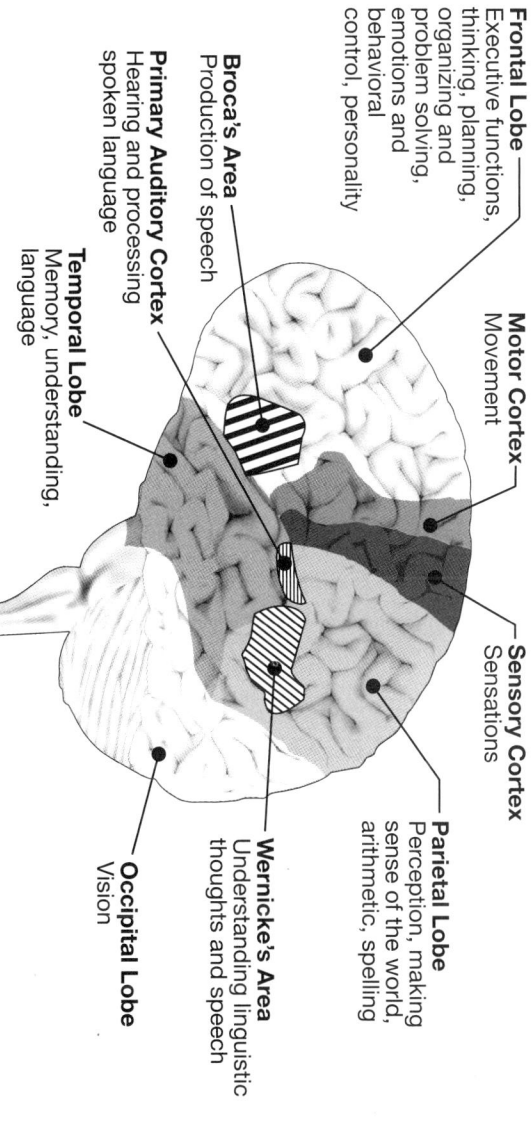

Frontal Lobe
Executive functions,
thinking, planning,
organizing and
problem solving,
emotions and
behavioral
control, personality

Broca's Area
Production of speech

Primary Auditory Cortex
Hearing and processing
spoken language

Temporal Lobe
Memory, understanding,
language

Motor Cortex
Movement

Sensory Cortex
Sensations

Parietal Lobe
Perception, making
sense of the world,
arithmetic, spelling

Wernicke's Area
Understanding linguistic
thoughts and speech

Occipital Lobe
Vision

FIGURE 1.4: *Brain areas for processing language and linguistic thought in relation to the major divisions of the cortex, also called the lobes of the brain.*

But, as a reminder that there is no separation between "mind" and "body," this description of the TPN shows that even our linguistic thoughts arise from living in a human body that senses the outside world via exteroception and the body's inner condition via interoception, proprioception, feelings that arise in the autonomic nervous system, and emotional feelings (see Table 1.2).

In early childhood, thoughts begin to form "in the head" around the age of four or five. Prior to that, as far as we know, children do not have narrative, linguistic thoughts. Thought originates in human development from what was originally spoken or signed speech that we learned to produce with the muscles of our mouth, tongue, throat, diaphragm and breath, and gestures of the arms, hands, body, and face.

All these motor movements that create speech are connected to the sensory and motor cortices of the brain and to Broca's area for speech production. The child's hearing and gradual understanding of speech sounds occur in the auditory senses, the auditory cortex, and the felt experience of the sounds of speech, tone of voice, and emotion carried in the voice of the person speaking.

Sometime around two and a half years of age, children begin to talk to themselves when they are not speaking with another person. This so-called private speech is a transitional developmental stage between talking to other people and TPN internal linguistic thinking. Children might talk to themselves out loud about an intended action ("I put that there"), describe an ongoing action ("Banging it"), make a statement to an object ("Get out of my way, chair!"), or ask a question and then answer it ("Why are you crying, Dolly? Because I'm sad").[12]

You can see how these examples of a young child's private speech are similar to TPN thoughts that involve explanations, reasons, and plans. Thought, in other words, originated as the embodied muscle movements of spoken language and the language of others that we heard via our auditory cortex and auditory sense organs in the ear, or written language that we read with our eyes and processed in the visual cortex in the brain's occipital lobe located at the back of the head (Figure 1.4). Jay Seitz, in an article entitled "The Bodily Basis of Thought," says, "We do not simply inhabit our bodies, we literally use them to think with."[13]

Keeping in mind that TPN thought is fundamentally embodied, let's consider an example. Suppose you spend a day or two feeling grouchy and easily irritated by something your partner or child or coworker says or does. You try to get on with your day by holding back this feeling, maybe "hearing" your TPN telling yourself that you are "just fine." Or maybe this feeling leaks out of you in speech with a somewhat nasty edge or tone that you know, almost instantly, you don't really mean because you can see how it hurts or affects others. You try to keep your head down and stay focused on your TPN thoughts about what you need to accomplish that day.

But what is really going on inside of you? For most people, the first and only strategy is to think about this question using your TPN. "Hmmm. Why am I so grouchy?" And then come the explanatory thoughts. Maybe it's that you haven't slept well? Maybe it is something someone said to you that was hurtful or annoying? Maybe you haven't been getting any down time or time for recreation? Maybe you are not getting enough loving attention or sexual intimacy with your partner? Maybe, maybe, maybe …

Sometimes such thought inquiries are helpful and sometimes they are not. What is the alternative? Talking to a trusted other (friend, partner, therapist) about your feelings might be helpful because another person who really listens to us also gives us permission to listen to ourselves. In this way, you might get closer to what your irritability is really trying to tell you, not in the language of words and sentences but in the language of felt experience.

The key is to simply let yourself feel the irritation, the annoyance, or whatever, and then your TPN can create thoughts and speech that are more honest and open: "I'm sorry I was so grouchy earlier. It must be what my boss said to me yesterday." Or "OK, I get it, I'm really upset about what you did earlier. It's not your fault, but it just rubbed me the wrong way."

These more honest explanations help, but it is also important to leave open the possibility that you won't get an answer that satisfies the thinking, TPN part of yourself. You won't be able to explain your way out of the problem. Sometimes just having a good cry is all that is needed. In chapter 3, we'll see why simply allowing our "real" or "deeper" feelings to emerge brings a sense of relief and restoration. We cry and we feel better and it can be just that simple. Present-moment felt experience, without any attempt at TPN mental understanding, can feel like a reawakening to our better selves.

You will find that, in general, the hit rate of "landing" into a present-moment felt experience beginning from a fast-moving focused thought train has pretty low odds. It wouldn't be wise to place any bets on the success of this route into felt experience. We can increase the odds by accepting that the "language" of felt experience is elusive because it is completely different from ordinary language and thought. The language of felt experience is composed of shifting, aimless, and mostly hidden emotions, sensations, and movements.

TPN thinking fools you into believing that you "know" (logically), or you think you know, what is going on with you. The disconcerting news is that your thinking self—full of ideas, compelling and addictive, often highly educated and intelligent—literally has *no idea* what you are really feeling! Felt experience is not an idea or a thought (see Table 1.1), and you can't arrive there by any logical, rational route.

Felt Experience vs. Default-Mode Thinking

In addition to the focused and purposeful thoughts of the TPN, another thinking part of the brain is called the *default-mode network* (DMN). The TPN involves thinking about things like the task or problem we are working on, or something about ourselves that we are attempting to understand, or self-help resources that we are searching the internet to find. The TPN is focused thinking while the DMN jumps around, as if it is picking up the bits and pieces of thought that got left behind by the insistent momentum of the TPN trying to get somewhere and figure out something.

The DMN produces thoughts that can be described as daydreaming, reviewing, rehashing, rehearsing, and mind-wandering—thoughts we think when we are off-task. Maybe DMN thought happens when we are going for a walk or exercising or resting or preparing food.

The DMN is the neural center for thoughts about social relationships in which we are a part, including empathic thinking (about what others may be feeling) and wondering about doing the "right" things with other people.[14] The DMN is activated when we have drifting thoughts about our body size and shape, our clothes, our looks, our personality (see discussion earlier in this chapter). But when we are simply being with our body experiences—without labeling or mentally commenting on them—the neural networks for felt experience (see Table 1.2 and descriptions throughout chapter 2) are more likely to be activated.[15] The DMN can also be a source for imagination of new ideas or creative thoughts that we can bring back into the TPN to process at a later time.

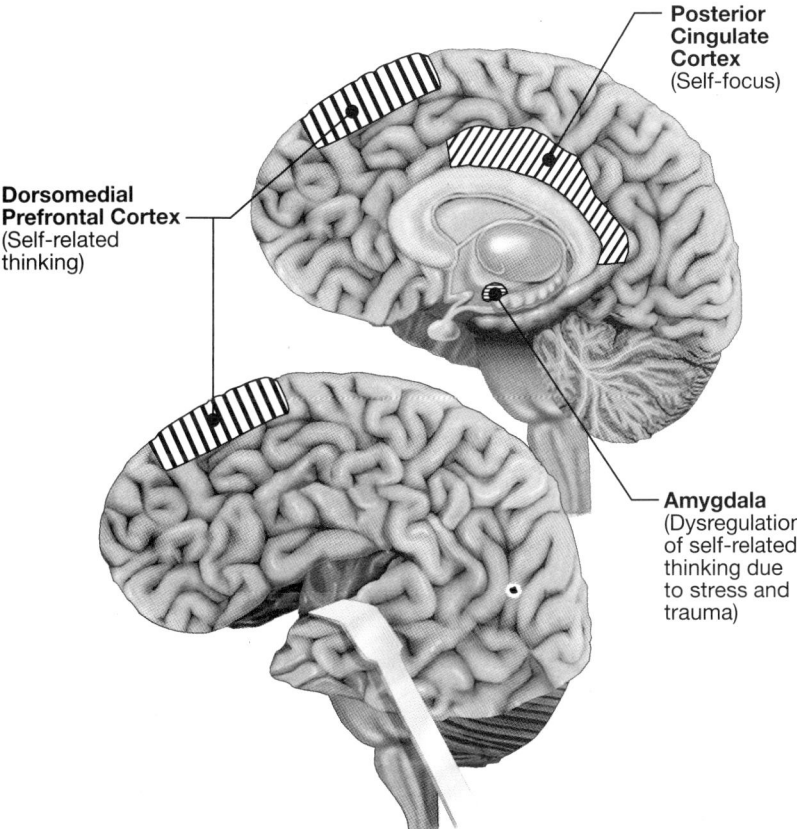

FIGURE 1.5: *The thinking brain: the default-mode network.*

One part of the DMN is the dorsomedial prefrontal cortex, which is deep in the frontal section of the brain, as shown in Figure 1.5 (compare this to the dors*olateral* prefrontal cortex on the outer layer of the frontal brain used to focus thoughts in the TPN, as shown in Figure 1.3). *Dorsal* means toward the top of the brain (as opposed to the ventral, or lower, part of the brain) and *medial* means toward the center of the brain (as opposed to the lateral, or outside, surface of the brain).

The dorsomedial prefrontal cortex responds to changes in serotonin, the neurotransmitter affecting self-related emotion and mood. The dorsolateral prefrontal cortex—the part of the TPN that helps us focus attention on a sight, sound, or task—responds instead to dopamine, which regulates information flow and how we allocate our attentional resources.[16]

The other part of the DMN is the posterior cingulate cortex. This brain area channels our DMN thoughts about the self. Notice that the TPN uses the anterior cingulate cortex (toward the front of the brain, emotion-related thoughts) while the DMN uses the posterior cingulate cortex (toward the back of the brain, self-related thoughts).

The imaginative and creative DMN thoughts typically occur when we are off-task and not worried about anything in particular. If, however, we are stressed about something or suffering from the aftereffects of some kind of trauma, the DMN can produce worried and anxious self-related thoughts that repeat sometimes endlessly in our heads, instead of the imaginative thinking described in the previous paragraphs.

This self-repetitive DMN thought is called *rumination*. This dysregulated aspect of the DMN is less like free-associative daydreaming and more like getting caught up in patterns of unproductive thoughts. We think or worry about defending our own point of view, either to ourselves or another person. There might be thoughts about things that were or might have been said that were harmful or hurtful to other people, or how we could have been more thoughtful and less irritable.[17]

Dysregulated DMN thoughts can also be about addictive cravings, such as for food, drugs, or sex; about not caring about anything; about risk taking and self-harming; or even about suicide. People who have suffered from a trauma are more likely to ruminate using words related to the traumatic event or to any kind of traumatic event that they might hear about from someone else or see in a movie or on TV.[18] Ruminative DMN thoughts occur when the amygdala (our fear- or threat-sensing part of the brain) gets activated and disrupts the free-flowing and creative communication between the dorsomedial prefrontal cortex and the posterior cingulate cortex (see Figure 1.5).

We learned earlier in this chapter that thinking and feeling are mutually exclusive, occurring in different brain networks. (The neural networks for thinking are illustrated in this chapter's figures, while those for feeling will be presented in chapter 2.) Just as thinking and feeling cannot occur simultaneously, activity in the TPN and DMN are also mutually exclusive. When our thoughts are composed of creative ideas, social actions, daydreams, and worries (the DMN), we cannot be focused on getting a task accomplished. When we are task focused with the TPN activated, we can't pay much attention to thinking about how best to respond to other people. Other people, when we are engaged in TPN thinking, are more likely to show up as strategic thoughts, such as how to best use others to collaborate on a project, or how to plan a party, or how to get someone into bed.[19]

The DMN is most active when you are done with the major tasks of your day, such as when you are lying in bed before falling asleep or when you wake up at night and thoughts are running around inside your head. Maybe you keep coming back in your thoughts to a particular encounter you had with another person. You keep replaying the conversation or shared experience, and maybe you think about how it might have been different or better. Or maybe it was a wonderful and inspiring conversation, and you keep thinking about the clever things you said or did, or how great you were in bed, or how witty you sounded at that dinner party. Or you picture the other person and remember how your remarks made them feel, replaying both your own role and your empathy for the other person.

The DMN is like a constant background, our verbal stream of consciousness. It is aptly named our *default state* because that is where our thoughts tend to go when we aren't working on anything in particular. It's not clear why, but people tend to be more secretive about their DMN thoughts, almost as if they are "felt" as private, personal musings and not for public consumption, or maybe somewhat embarrassing when held up to the light of shared experience.

When we want to "turn off" thinking in order to access felt experience, we are swimming upstream against both the TPN and the DMN. That's why accessing felt experience directly takes practice and why it almost always requires the help of another person. This might mean working with a teacher in an ESA practice, or individually with a therapist who is trained in ESA, or being in the company of a trusted other person who is willing to just be present with you and allow you space to come closer to your feelings.

As you go through this book, your TPN will find some satisfaction in understanding why felt experience is so elusive and also critically important for making choices about work, health, and relationships. Your DMN might have reason to congratulate yourself or beat yourself up for staying with or avoiding your felt experiences. In chapters 3, 4, and 5 you will have the chance to learn how to be more aware of when you are thinking or when you are actually feeling yourself, based on many concrete examples from everyday life.

Intelligence vs. Embodiment

People say that what we are all seeking is a meaning for life. I don't think that's what we're really seeking. I think that what we're really seeking is an experience of being alive so that our life experience on the purely physical plane will have resonances within our innermost being and reality so that we actually feel the rapture of being alive.

—JOSEPH CAMPBELL, *THE POWER OF MYTH*[20]

For those of us raised in societies with formal systems of education, we learned how to *make meaning* of ourselves by using our powerful tools of TPN and DMN thought. We developed thinking tools to try to understand ourselves and others or find the answers to our problems and preoccupations. This is because formal education in schools generally emphasizes building intelligence via the TPN's focused and regulated thinking, speaking, and writing.

Then we spend the rest of our waking moments rehashing and rehearsing all of that in our DMN. Cultural practices such as social networking have—like formal education for the TPN—supported, indulged, and developed the DMN as our go-to off-task activity. Our devices and social practices in Western society are primarily and almost totally devoted to thinking, writing, explaining.

Even when we're sending photos and emojis, our intention is to express a thought to the receiver. That smiley face you sent might make your recipient smile, and it might come from something that made you happy, but if you really paid attention to your process of sending and receiving, you would most likely find it filled with thoughts. The feelings may be real, but they would be fleeting moments in the ongoing flow of thought and verbal discourse: "Hmm, I wonder just which one of these emojis is the best way to convey my feeling?"

If this description of your texting practices seems cynical, then take some time during your texting episode to slow down and monitor yourself. When you took and sent that photo, did it move you to tears or into a state of relief and the absence of thought? Or were you thinking about the quality of the photo, how you looked in it, or whether it conveyed what you "wanted" to say? Did you accompany the photo with explanatory text, just to make sure you got your point across? Were you thinking about how it would be received and how you might respond?

In this little experiential exercise, you needn't be judgmental. It's only about observing that thinking is lurking around even when you are ostensibly communicating about feelings. Of course, you might become judgmental about how you get trapped into thinking. Notice if your DMN worries about self-presentation and self-evaluation kick in. See if you can just observe all of that right now in order to mark it as a kind of baseline of how you are generally operating in relation to people and things. Maybe, by the end of this book, your baseline will shift from being mostly in your head toward being someplace in your body that is closer to your heart?

Because of the need to score higher on standardized tests in order to receive federal funding that promotes academic performance, schools in the United States have severely curtailed or eliminated physical education and performing arts programming, the disciplines that might promote the development of the felt-experience component of ESA. In order to learn thinking skills, it is believed, children should sit still, keep quiet, obey instructions, and the like. This takes a toll on the body. Children often endure sitting for long hours, not being able to move or stretch or go to the bathroom when needed. They are expected to know how to "behave" in these ways and are likely censured if they do not.[21]

This assumption that guides formal educational planning is, however, ultimately counterproductive. Thought processes—what standardized tests are supposedly assessing—are part of embodiment, and they will become constricted in a constricted body. Even when children have an opportunity to move in their free time, they are likely to avoid it: vegging out in front of a video display or doing some of that TPN-based texting on a mobile device seems easier because thinking is easy, always there, our constant companion.

The price paid for ignoring the body—its movements and senses—is the festering of physical and mental disease and dysfunction. Hence the current epidemic of childhood obesity, eating disorders, diabetes, attention deficit hyperactivity disorder (ADHD), depression and anxiety, and lack of physical fitness.

If you think mental processes are independent of body function (mind vs. body!), think again. Children need to move their bodies in order to learn. Most children fidget during cognitive tasks when they are required to sit still at their desks, and children diagnosed with ADHD move around even more. These movements, contrary to what one might expect, actually improve children's ability to learn and to remember. Researchers, therefore, do not recommend interventions to reduce body movement. They promote the surprising and counterintuitive idea of letting kids wiggle and move about during class.[22] Why not have bouncy balls for sitting and yoga mats for lying down during class?

Preschool children who were enrolled in a creative dance movement program as part of their Head Start experience had greater gains in social competence and more reductions in behavior problems than children who were given a TPN-based program of learning to control attention that did not include a component of movement and felt experience.[23] Elementary school children who took physical education classes requiring vigorous activity that met the Healthy People guidelines had better grades than children who did not.[24] The Healthy People guidelines, developed by the US Department of

Health and Human Services, suggest that moderate activity should be thirty minutes per day for at least five days per week. For those doing vigorous activity, twenty minutes per day for at least three days per week is sufficient to meet the criteria.

Middle and high school students who are more physically active have a considerably lower risk of depression and anxiety.[25] It turns out that during middle and high school, students can be sedentary for up to nine hours a day, and that only counts the time they spend at school! This is due to sitting in classes, increased use of smart devices, and lack of opportunities to exercise. University students who are more physically active have enhanced memory and thinking skills compared to those students who are less active.[26]

Yoga, tai chi, and meditation training for children has effects similar to vigorous exercise. Children diagnosed with ADHD, especially, are able to reduce their anxiety, concentrate better in school, and have less interpersonal conflict after only six weeks of regular yoga or meditation.[27] Anything that enhances embodiment via felt experience is likely to have the same or similar effects.

Why does exercise enhance felt experience? During vigorous aerobic activity—defined as an intensity that causes sweating and puffing—different parts of your body will speak to you as needed, and you have to listen. You might notice that you are having difficulty breathing, or that your exertion is creating fatigue and possibly muscular pains. You might notice that your feet or hands hurt, or that sweat is stinging your eyes. When you exercise, you have an opportunity to let your body speak to you in a way that is similar to the experiential exercise introduced earlier: by letting your attention float around to wherever your body is calling it.

You might think that high-achieving athletes, dancers, and other performance artists are able to ignore their body aches and pains by pushing through them, suppressing the felt experience, and focusing on the outcome or goal. In fact, the professionals who ignore their bodies end up suffering from injury and burnout. The best athletes and performance artists can monitor their ESA across multiple levels of awareness, everything from aches and pains to endurance, to emotional feelings of excitement or discouragement, to negative thought patterns that might get in the way of functioning at their highest level.

Runners who score higher on tests of interoception, for example, are more efficient physiologically: they use less oxygen, run faster, and have less muscle tension.[28] Children who are taught to pay attention to their body senses during physical education classes and after-school recreational sports have better grades and test scores in school and are more effective in social relationships.[29]

Restorative natural environments are an especially important means of enhancing felt experience in children and adults, and most especially for those who suffer from the effects of stress and trauma. With increasing urbanization, the opportunities for people to freely contact the natural world are becoming more limited. This has been called "nature-deficit disorder"[30] and has led to recommendations for more outdoor activities. Being outside in nature enhances and expands our fully embodied selves, puts our worries in perspective, calms the mind, and soothes the spirit.

Access to green areas such as playgrounds, parks, and nearby countryside enhances cognitive functioning, reduces stress, improves sensory and motor skills, and ameliorates the symptoms of ADHD in children.[31] The body is alive and well when people are getting hands dirty, smelling plants, running through grass, climbing trees, walking in the surf, listening to birds, and watching the clouds roll by or the stars twinkle.

Even if children can't regularly be in a natural environment, one of the most accessible ways for children and even adults to contact nature is through animals. Animals have a special appeal to children, who love pretending to be an animal, imitating animal movements and sounds, playing with and cuddling pets, and going to zoos and farms.

Gail Melson, in a book called *Why the Wild Things Are: Animals in the Lives of Children*, describes research showing that these encounters enhance self-awareness and interoception.[32] Children who pretend to be a turtle, for example, know that they are not a turtle, which then encourages an awareness of their own body and how it differs from the animal's. Yet, at the same time, children aren't merely thinking about a turtle but rather *becoming* the turtle in a fundamentally embodied way by getting on all fours, putting a cover over their body, stretching and contracting their neck, arms, and legs, and so on.

We could all use a dose of being more childlike to enhance our felt experience and subsequent well-being. Our perception of adult responsibilities may not permit such indulgence. But there are new research findings that build on these ideas, like showing that more than eight out of every ten disadvantaged preschoolers from two urban areas showed significant developmental delays in basic motor skills such as running, jumping, throwing, and catching. Children actually need to be trained in athletics, dance, music, and other motor activities. Like learning a language, all motor skill learning requires instruction and feedback.[33]

In Western culture, we've operated for centuries under the assumption that the body's "lower" needs and urges must be suppressed in order to develop our "higher" human faculties of thought, intelligence, and moral behavior (mind vs. body!). It is time to wash our collective hands of this cruel dichotomy that has abandoned the poor self-regulators and those with disabilities prey to feelings of shame and worthlessness, not to mention lost opportunities to achieve their fullest potential.[34]

Felt Experience Is Compromised by Stress and Trauma

Conditions such as trauma, illness, medical challenges, family and work stress, and other unresolved life experiences lead us to become disconnected from present-moment felt experience. On the other hand, when we can truly listen to ourselves, it shifts our whole neurophysiology; we relax, and parts of the nervous system are activated that promote restoration and repair throughout the body. Research has shown that sustained access to our felt experience can revise and reprogram neural circuits that have developed persistent post-traumatic dysfunction, significantly boost the effects of medical, pharmacological, psychological, and complementary and alternative interventions, and open the way to profound change in our inner and outer lives.[35]

As explained in the next chapter, felt experience is supported by a dedicated network of nerve cells and connections within the brain and body. This network is different from the TPN and DMN networks that support thinking.

The felt experience of our body in health and illness is necessary for the nervous system to locate in the body the sources of dis-ease and direct the body's own resources to facilitate healing. When your health care provider asks you, "Where does it hurt?" or "What are you feeling in your belly (or chest, or head, or wherever)?" then you need to access your felt experience to provide some guidance to your care provider in finding the best treatment.

If we can't sense that our body is in pain or that we are close to burnout because of stressful life conditions, then we can't take steps to modulate the stress or seek help from medical or behavioral health providers. This impairment in felt experience means that we will be less likely to avoid or to alleviate potentially more serious health risks.

But impaired felt experience can also contribute to impairing a healthy physiological balance in all body systems. In other words, it is not just that impaired felt experience makes us avoid our feelings of illness or distress so we can't notice or talk about them. *Impaired felt experience actually makes our condition worse.*

As one example, when we are under stress and we ignore it or can't sense how that stress may be affecting our body, the stress detector in our brain (the amygdala) will dampen our felt experience. This is because in challenging conditions of survival under threat or stress, we can't afford to devote energy to feeling ourselves. The amygdala diminishes felt experience while amplifying the TPN and altering the DMN as ways of coping with the current situation.

Sure, when we have a lot of work or family demands, we might have a dim sense that we are exhausted or on the edge of catching a cold or having a headache. But our powerful survival system keeps us going, thinking, doing, staying awake at night, doing more, overdoing, pushing ourselves to meet external demands or demands that we place on ourselves because of some expectation that we should be doing even more. We think we should be a better parent, a more loving spouse, or a more productive employee, or get better grades in school, or make the team, or whatever (probably unrealistic) expectations we place on ourselves.

This pushing ourselves can only happen if our amygdala—while concurrently turning down our sensitivity to interoceptive feelings—sends signals to the hypothalamus and pituitary to secrete ACTH into the blood in order to promote the secretion of cortisol from the adrenal glands into the blood (see Figure 1.2, p. 5). Cortisol is the main hormone produced under conditions of stress and trauma because, as explained earlier in this chapter, it is a blood sugar that provides energy for responding to the real or perceived stressors.

But if the source of stress persists (like being in a dysfunctional family where we don't feel supported or may suffer abuse, or working a difficult job with long hours and low pay, or having a demanding school workload and exams that we cannot change), then cortisol will continue to be produced. Excess cortisol can actually alter brain function, making us feel stressed even after the stressor is no longer present. In addition, excessive cortisol arising from ongoing stressful conditions can alter the function of the immune system by creating states of inflammation in the body.[36]

Inflammation, like the redness that appears around a recent wound on the skin, is a first-aid response of the immune system. The inflammation from a superficial wound leads to swelling and redness and the creation of pus to expel any irritants. If all goes well, inflammatory cell production soon slows down, and the immune system begins to send repair cells that create scabs to cover and close the wound and eventually regenerate torn skin tissue and reattach broken blood vessels.

When we are under the kinds of psychological stress discussed previously, *inflammatory immune cells are sent to all the organ systems* that are working harder to cope with the excess demands, such as the heart and blood vessels, the lungs and respiratory tissues, and the digestive system. This is all good in the short term.

We might tax our cardiovascular and respiratory and muscular systems with excessive hard work or exercise, but then, hopefully, we can slow down and rest so that the immune repair cells can rebuild tissues in those organs. This is actually how we can build cardiovascular fitness (by breaking down worn tissues and rebuilding stronger ones) or how we can develop stress resilience. Resilience comes from successfully coping with a stressor and then taking time to rest and recover, which rebuilds and strengthens neural pathways for handling more challenging tasks as well as supporting neural pathways for taking the time to sleep, let down, and recharge our batteries.

Stress is potentially toxic if our felt experience is impaired, and we can't sense that our body is under stress, and we can't sense that we need down time. In these conditions, *the inflammation will become chronic (it continues and there is no repair) without our being aware that our vital organ systems are in a nearly constant state of being wounded.* Without awareness and without preventive and restorative practices that arise from that awareness, the stress-induced inflammation will ultimately lead to illness conditions including sickness behaviors and fatigue, depression, eating disorders, insomnia, anxiety, and a host of possible physical ailments.[37]

We need to give recovery due respect and give ourselves the opportunity to heal without overdoing, overthinking, or pushing ourselves beyond our limits.[38] Treatments to minimize the effects of trauma and stress by enhancing embodied felt experience have been shown to improve many different types of mental and physical illness conditions.

Resilience is a concept that refers to one's ability to adapt to stress, trauma, and adversity by using appropriate cognitive, emotional, and physiological resources. This might include staying on task to find the help we need, accepting medical and emotional support in times of crises, or developing a wellness, rest, and recovery plan. Once we are out of danger and moving toward recovery, resilience also shows up as conservation of emotional and physiological resources.

People who are low on resilience are less likely to regain normal function following stressful injury or illness situations. They stay in a stress state, which shows up as dysregulated DMN worry or guilt and the TPN pushing them beyond their limits.[39] Workers who were less resilient, for example, found it more difficult to modulate unwanted ruminations when they were under pressure to complete a task in a short time. More resilient workers, on the other hand, were able to modulate their thinking even with increased time pressure.[40]

In one research study done at the University of California, San Diego (USA), for example, activity in the felt experience areas of the brain was compared between individuals with low resilience vs. high resilience. Supporting the theme of this book that felt experience is essential to well-being and health, low-resilience individuals in this study were also low on their ability to access their felt experience; they were less able to feel the effects and aftereffects of stress and illness.[41]

People who have experienced early-life stress, early-life trauma, or later-life trauma are less likely to be resilient in the face of everyday stress.[42] Early-life trauma especially is a risk factor for depression, post-traumatic stress disorder (PTSD), ADHD, anxiety, substance abuse, and physical diseases such as diabetes, heart disease, and immune function disorders.[43]

Think about this: Some of us, maybe all of us at times, can become impaired or actively avoid the felt experiences related to how our bodies may be compromised. We tend to ignore pain, deny our own vulnerabilities and fragilities, or act like our physical and emotional wounds are of no concern. Probably, most of us do this at times when demands are high.

What we need to understand is that *ignoring the signals from the body in order to get on with whatever we think we should be getting on with is not a route to getting better*. With these denials, we are more likely to get reinjured or fall into a more serious illness state, more likely to put more stress and strain on our body, and risk compromising our ability to recover and heal.

What is particularly striking is that in low-resilience individuals, *the brain regions related to felt experience* (the insula and thalamus; see Figures 2.2, p. 53, and 2.3, p. 62) *were activated even though this activation did not register in their conscious awareness as a felt experience*. This means that for low-resilience individuals, their brain continues to produce signals related to distressed feelings, pain, and higher physiological arousal. Instead of being channeled into feeling, these neural impulses are rerouted into TPN and DMN thinking.

The authors of this research from the University of California, San Diego, on people who show high vs. low resilience recommend

> bodily awareness training as potential interventions for those who report impaired stress resilience ... low resilient individuals may not be effectively using information from the moment, which may lead to impaired decision making in the presence of stressful environments.[44]

Other recent research testifies to the general conclusion that impaired felt experience is related to chronic states of anxiety, depression, inflammation in the immune system that can lead to both mental and physical illnesses, thought and memory impairments, obesity, and in general, multiple forms of mental and physical illness.[45] This list includes cardiovascular disease, high blood pressure, gastrointestinal diseases such as colitis and ulcers, autoimmune disorders including cancers, persistent muscle pain, and respiratory diseases such as asthma.[46]

The reverse is also true: illness and impaired immune function suppress and alter normal felt experience, emotional expression, and emotional well-being.[47] If we suffer from a condition like chronic depression or anxiety, it is particularly challenging to our ability to sustain felt experience (i.e., to escape from ruminative DMN thoughts), and therefore particularly important to work at maintaining that felt experience when anxious or depressed. Kara Baskin, a journalist for the *Boston Globe* who has a diagnosed anxiety disorder, writes that

> the only way out is by sitting with the discomfort until it dissipates. Acknowledge that you're scared, and then tell yourself that you'll breathe, and you'll exist—yes, you will exist, minute by minute— until the feeling goes away. It's the most un-American thing ever, yet: You must sometimes feel bad. [Anxiety] will continue to bounce on your shoulders like a thorny goblin until you grab it, stare it in the face, and have a firm chat.[48]

The "chat" Baskin seems to be referring to is a conversation with the body in the language of felt experience and not the focused language of the TPN. Access to the language of felt experience is important in itself because it attunes us to ourselves, which is intrinsically rewarding and ultimately calming. Felt experience—even the felt experience of pain or anxiety—just feels good because it settles the nervous system and gives us the confidence that we are grounded in the reality of the body.

Summary and Conclusions: Loss and Restoration of Our Embodied Selves

So, as individuals and as a culture, it seems that we have gotten ourselves into a situation where our ability to access our felt experience is compromised and impaired. Most of us, if we are honest with ourselves, don't heed Kara Baskin's advice. We don't take the time to pay sufficient attention to the internal condition of our body. We don't slow down to feel ourselves in a way that might bring some sense of ease or relief. Our felt experience may seem lost to us at certain times in our lives, but the message of this book is that we always have the possibility to rediscover it—and this is perhaps the most helpful form of self-care that we can take.

My own personal experience, and my experience as an ESA practitioner who helps people find their way back to themselves, leads me to the conclusion that most of us need help in finding a way back into this mysterious and nonlogical realm of felt experience. It takes practice, guidance, and even courage to step out of our habits of doing and thinking. Most of us need help and support for stress reduction and for the resolution of old trauma states.

This book is about the *restoration* of our lost felt experience. There are several meanings of this word, restoration. One meaning is the recovery of the ability to access felt experiences that had been lost or hidden. Another meaning is that fully accessing felt experience in the present moment without intervening thought is fundamentally healing.

Being fully "in" our felt experiences is restorative because it can lead to a sense of relief, peace, and relaxation. When we enter this kind of state, it allows all our functional systems (respiratory, cardiovascular, hormonal, digestive, sexual-reproductive, neurophysiological, and immune functions) to activate cellular repair processes that promote whole-body health.[49]

One of the reasons this book contains a lot of information about anatomy and physiology is in order to make clear that our bodies have dedicated neural networks for feeling into ourselves and for thinking about and understanding ourselves. Our bodies are built in such a way that thinking and feeling are essential components of human function, just as much life-maintaining as our hearts beating and our breath flowing.

Fortunately, Western health care practices are changing. "Mental" illnesses are no longer seen as entirely "in the head," and physicians often prescribe an individualized combination of medication and psychotherapy for effective treatment. More medical centers and insurance companies are providing clinics and resources related to healthy lifestyle practices such as nutrition and exercise and to whole-person practices such as psychotherapy, massage, acupuncture, meditation, yoga, tai chi, and other body-awareness disciplines.

Fortunately, there is now a large amount of respected scientific research on the health effects of many of these "alternative and complementary" practices. This book is not intended to promote any particular practice because each person has unique needs and comfort zones from which they may be willing to explore alternative health care that promotes a greater sense of ease and safety in staying in the present moment with their felt experiences. Nor is this book intended to be a manifesto to make the case for the importance of embodiment practices. There are now many books and resources on these important topics.

The purpose of this book is to introduce the new idea that there are three primary ways in which we can experience ourselves: dysregulated, modulated, and restorative embodied self-awareness. These three "states" of ESA will be introduced in the next chapter. This book is meant as a resource for you to learn about these three states, both how to think about them as they apply to yourself and the people around you and how to feel them in your everyday life. You can use your awareness of each of these three states as a way to navigate through life, to better assess the states in which you are living at any given moment, and to find resources that may help you out of being lost in dysregulated ESA and into becoming more whole and healthy in modulated and restorative ESA.

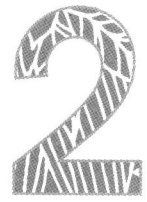

Three States of Embodied Self-Awareness and Four Forms of Felt Experience

This chapter provides an introductory explanation of a new way of understanding embodied self-awareness that is composed of three distinct and mutually exclusive states: restorative, modulated, and dysregulated embodied self-awareness.[1] As we'll see, each state has a unique pattern of felt experience and thinking that describes three unique ways in which we can experience living in a human body. In the previous chapter, we covered the forms of thinking that can occur in each state of ESA. In this chapter, we'll discuss the four different types of felt experience—interoceptive, proprioceptive, autonomic, and emotional—that can occur in each of these three states of ESA.

Dividing ESA into three different states has a number of implications. One implication is that we can only be in one of these states at any given time. We can experience ourselves as dysregulated or modulated, for example, but not both at once. A second implication is that it becomes important to learn to distinguish the state in which we are living at any particular moment. This chapter provides an introduction to the specific forms of thinking and feeling that uniquely define each state of ESA. Chapter 3 will take us into more details of the forms of thinking and feeling in each state.

This leads to the third implication of the three-state picture of ESA: our state of ESA can shift and change. We don't stay in any one of these states forever. Tracking the changes from one to another state can become part of our embodied self-awareness. What times or places or situations predispose us to be in one or another state? What helps us move away from dysregulated ESA and into more productive modulated ESA or more soothing restorative ESA? Chapters 4, 5, and 6 give examples and ways of facilitating these state changes in ourselves.

The Three States of Embodied Self-Awareness

At the end of the previous chapter, the idea of restoration was introduced, so let's begin with a brief overview of the state of **restorative embodied self-awareness**. This state is primarily about felt experience rather than thought. The felt experience in this state is *always* accompanied by real, observable changes of the physical body *coming to rest*: a deeper breath, a softening of the muscles or posture, a felt sense of relaxation, or the kind of crying in which we feel genuinely touched, perhaps cleansed, and that evokes a sense of a deeper truth beyond words.

This relaxation is the primary indicator of being in a state of restorative ESA. So, if you don't feel this physiological shift into a sense of greater ease, then you are more likely to be in a state of modulated or dysregulated ESA.

As discussed at the end of chapter 1, coming into a state of restorative ESA can be profoundly healing. There is a kind of wonder in spontaneously (with diffuse attention and without thinking or planning) arriving at a genuine feeling. This might be the experience of suddenly being overwhelmed with joy or sadness. Tears in the middle of an ordinary day, for example, may come unexpectedly and overcome someone who has recently lost a person close to them. This moment of grieving may happen because of a memory that emerges from doing something that we had previously done with that person. The tears and sadness become restorative when we can let the feeling just arise in us, experience it fully, and let it pass in a way that provides a sense of relief. We don't have to explain it or understand it. Restorative ESA is more about acceptance, about allowing ourselves to be overcome with a feeling and just being present in that moment with whatever comes up.

Alternatively, restorative ESA could manifest as a moment of awe in front of a work of art, in the presence of great natural beauty, or when having a deep spiritual experience.[2] These kinds of moments activate a cascade of hormones and neurotransmitters that bring us into a place of softness, tenderness, and vulnerability: a place from which there is no need to do anything else, no need to use our TPN (task-positive network) or DMN (default-mode network) to solve any problems, no compulsion to work on something or to figure it out. Rather, we just allow ourselves to feel tingly or warm or astounded.

Restorative ESA sometimes comes with thoughts as well as feelings. Restorative ESA thoughts are typically images, sounds, vivid memories, or simple words that resonate with and amplify the felt experience. In the example of grief, it could be a memory of the face of the person who died or a situation you experienced with that person. This thought is like a picture or even a short video, but there is no narration, no story that goes with it. Somehow, you just immediately recognize that image, and it evokes and amplifies spontaneous crying and feelings of sadness or longing.

While sitting or walking in the mountains or by the seashore, or standing in front of a work of art, or listening to music, or watching a dance or musical performance, that feeling of awe might go along with a few words like *amazing* or *incredible*. Those few simple words somehow expand or acknowledge for you the felt experience of being overcome, or a sense of oneness with something vast and incomprehensible. Some forms of stirring classical music, such as Mozart's *Requiem*, are more likely to evoke chills and goose bumps connected with awe compared with music that stirs people to dance and move. The latter evokes a modulated sympathetic state of enjoyment, while the former evokes a parasympathetic restorative state.[3]

After having one of these restorative experiences, maybe you begin to use your TPN to think about it. You might think about a story related to your lost loved one, and if you are with someone, you might feel compelled to tell the story or to explain why you were so suddenly taken by your emotion. Similarly, in that place of natural beauty and after the moment of restorative awe has passed, you might want to compare it to other places you have visited, to yourself or with your companions. You might want to come up with some way to understand why this place is so special to you.

We learned in chapter 1 that when we are thinking, we cannot at the same time be with our felt experience. So whenever streams of logical thought—even thoughts about a very recent restorative experience—come into our awareness, they take us out of the restorative state. Logical thoughts are those composed of sentences, stories, or narratives. The thoughts can be productive and goal-oriented, those that come from the TPN. Or they can be more creative, daydreamy, or meandering thoughts that arise in the DMN in this particular special place.

These thoughts that occur inside of us, or that we share verbally with others, may become an important part of our experience. They may provide a meaning and context to that experience. Still, when our TPN or DMN is being engaged, we can no longer access what was, just moments ago, the actual felt experience of grief or awe. The thinking has shifted us into a state of **modulated embodied self-awareness.**

In modulated ESA, rather than simply being in the moment of felt experience, we are giving ourselves an explanation or making sense of an experience. Other examples of this kind of TPN thought are trying to envision the route we have to take to get to a particular location, imagining an upcoming romantic encounter and how we might want it to unfold, or picturing in images a dance or sports movement pattern that we plan to do or to teach to others.

Modulated ESA has two important benefits. First, because modulated ESA is primarily composed of thought, it gives us an opportunity to explain and understand, to get insights, and to plan and move forward. Second, the concept of modulated means that we can indulge in such thoughts but are not stuck in them. We can slow down—at least for a brief period of time—and reconnect with our felt experience.

Modulated means that we can adjust, regulate, self-monitor, or self-control our thinking in such a way that we can be productive; it also means that we can take a break to give ourselves time to recharge our batteries, to rest, or to nourish ourselves in some way. Modulated means that we have the potential to alternate felt experience with thinking. In modulated ESA, however, TPN and DMN thinking or speaking is the main attraction, while felt experience is a short or transient break from the ongoing task-oriented activity.

Suppose you are busy and occupied with completing a task—getting something done at work, or making a meal, or playing with your children. Your TPN is guiding you in this activity with focus and goal direction. At some point during this activity, you might suddenly sense that you are losing the ability to concentrate, or that there is an ache in your neck or back, or that you are hungry or thirsty or need to go to the bathroom.

At this point, your body is sending you a text message: "I can't concentrate anymore. I can't sit like this because it hurts. I need to pee (or get a drink, or something to eat)." Modulated ESA means that we can actually "read" the text message and stop the activity so that we can take that break and refresh ourselves. In so doing, we may have some brief moments of felt experience, like a breath of fresh air or rubbing our shoulders or lower back and feeling the ache, or feeling the relief of relieving ourselves, the taste of a drink or snack, or being uplifted by checking in with someone we love.

Modulated also means that after we take this break, we come back to the activity more refreshed and can keep pursuing our plans and goals. The break we took was like answering the body's text message with another text: "OK, you're right, I needed to take a break, but now it's time to get back to work." The break is brief and provides the needed respite, but it is just another text message. It is not like dropping what you are doing and finding a quiet and safe place where you can sink into a more fully restorative ESA state.

Or maybe you decide to do something that takes more time, like go for a walk or a run or lie down to rest, or whatever you feel your body needs. Maybe that takes an hour, more like a phone conversation than a text message. Most of the time, for most of us who are busy with many things, these activities that give us a longer break from our goals will typically be filled with DMN-type thoughts.

Even though this thinking is more aimless and nondirected, it is still composed of focused and narrative thought. Maybe some new and creative ideas will come to us when we are off-task, ideas that we can bring back to the problem we were working on. Maybe we will rehearse and plan the next steps of the day. Maybe we will remember to say something to another person or send that birthday card.

These kinds of modulated DMN thoughts are helpful in bringing us more in touch with ourselves and with others. It is as if our thoughts, once they are not engaged with a task, can "spread out" and pick up shards of many different activities that occupy our work, family, and leisure time. Using the word *modulated* for this kind of useful DMN thought suggests not only that it serves an important purpose in encompassing the fullness of our lives but also that we potentially have the ability to stop these thoughts and access our felt experience. Modulated felt experience, however, is different from restorative felt experience. The former is relatively brief while the latter is more long-lasting.

Feeling, expressing, and disclosing emotions and body sensations, even for a short time in modulated ESA, can often lead to effective and healthy changes. Modulated ESA can help us make sense of at least some of our feelings and symptomatic sensations like pain and fatigue, and this making-sense leads to the possibility of adopting health-promoting practices and seeking appropriate support.

Modulated felt experience can allow a short break that wakes up the body and alerts us to any aches or pains, feelings of accomplishment or disappointment, or times of shared laughter or tears with another person. These brief felt experiences happen as part of the flow of an ongoing task. Restorative felt experience is radically different: it reaches into what seems like the core of our being, alters our physiology into a state of relaxation, and can only occur when we completely let go of doing things and thinking about things.

As we saw in chapter 1, the DMN can also create thoughts that are unproductive and not at all creative: "Why am I so sad? Am I sick or just lazy? Does my life really matter to anyone?" These types of thoughts are typically self-centered and ruminative—that is, they repeat many times and it seems like we cannot turn them off.

This kind of DMN thinking is part of the third kind of ESA, called **dysregulated embodied self-awareness**. In modulated ESA, we can stop our thoughts and take a moment to feel what is happening in our body. We may not completely settle into a state of restorative relaxation, but being modulated means that if we can take at least a short break, and if we had the time and space, we could choose to access our restorative ESA.

When we are in a state of dysregulated ESA, we may have felt experiences in addition to ruminative thinking. Dysregulated felt experiences are very different from the felt experiences in restorative and modulated ESA. Dysregulated felt experiences include chronic pain, addictive urges, anxiety, depression, worthlessness, shame, risk taking, and self-doubt.

Dysregulated is the sense that we are *stuck* in these thoughts and feelings that we cannot modulate. We can't escape. We stay in states of anxiety or depression; we can feel angry or irritated that these feelings just simmer in the background and don't go away. We may be easily provoked to attack or to judge others.

When we're dysregulated, if these thoughts and feelings become too much to handle and we can't slow them down and modulate, then our body turns to a protective survival mechanism called *dissociation* or *freeze*. This means that we can go numb or feel confused, disconnected, or detached from ourselves. Dysregulated ESA is what was described in chapter 1 as an impairment in felt experience that shifts whole-body physiological function in ways that can promote serious mental and physical disease states.

Summarizing and Comparing the Three States

Modulated ESA occurs when thoughts are more productive—like finding strategies to slow down, meditate, eat better, get more sleep, exercise, spend more time with loved ones, solve problems at home and work. Restorative ESA states are relatively rare, which means that in our daily lives we are most likely to be in states of either modulated or dysregulated ESA. Reprising one of the themes of chapter 1, restorative ESA takes time, it takes practice, it takes a commitment to ourselves, and it usually takes getting the right kind of help or training.

Modulated ESA is a state that is essential to being productive and carrying on a normal social and work life. The ability to stay focused on a task, to allow our DMN to come up with new ideas and helpful reminders when we are off-task, and to take breaks and access felt experiences keeps us going and allows us to accomplish our life goals.

But modulated ESA has a hidden danger. This state can be deceptive because it captivates our attention so fully that *we think* we are in the best place ever. What actually happens is that when we start to feel something, *we think* we know what is going on in our felt experience. Our TPN jumps right in and tries to classify and explain: "I must feel tired or hungry," or "I probably am a little annoyed at you," or "I did a great job there and I'm proud of myself."

These kinds of thoughts are deceptive because they come from off-the-shelf cultural categories that seem to explain our feelings or our expectations for ourselves or other people. These thoughts are shaped, however, by our developmental and sociocultural histories. Sometimes these thoughts are just plain nonsense, a story we make up that has the effect of hiding a deeper feeling from ourselves or from other people.

If we really let ourselves feel our tiredness, we might discover a depth of exhaustion and burnout that would force us to confront some difficult choices about our life and goals. If we settled into the feeling of annoyance, we might find that we are almost overwhelmingly lonely and in need of intimacy and meaningful interpersonal connection that may not be happening for us in the moment. If we spent time feeling our sense of pride, we might find that we are not getting the support and encouragement we are longing for.

Each time that we take sufficient time to settle into a felt experience—even the painful and challenging experiences just mentioned—we have the possibility to enter into a state of restorative ESA. This is because our nervous system seems to be wired in a way that activates relaxation when we finally allow ourselves to just feel something. When we drop our dys-regulated defenses and our modulated justifications, there is a sudden and unexpected sense of relief as the truth of our felt experience is allowed to wash over us.

In thought, we can make it up as we go along and convince ourselves that we are right or wrong. This form of conceptual self-awareness is a kind of "false" self, false because when thinking, we are fundamentally cut off from whatever we might actually feel. Our "real" or "true" selves—the messages from our felt experiences—remain hidden behind the culturally constructed conceptual self (see pp. 84–85).

In modulated ESA, we only catch the outlines of felt experience because we then quickly move on to the go-to explanations, the to-do list, the next task. We *know* we are working too hard, so it *makes sense* to commit to taking yoga or meditation classes, to see a private practitioner who can support ESA awareness, to eat and sleep better, to taking the time for ourselves in everyday life to practice slowing down. Doing these things helps, right? Maybe.

For most of us, these classes and practices activate in us the same cultural strategies that we learned growing up, going to school, and at work. We learned how to think, to achieve, to meet goals and expectations. The body-awareness practices we learn in yoga, meditation, tai chi, and many other disciplines make sense to our TPN because they can indeed help us modulate and feel better, and this book will review lots of good science to support this outcome. Just plain old aerobic exercise can have the effect of modulating negative mood states, making us feel more alive, giving us new energy and a more positive outlook. When we feel down, tired, impatient, or unproductive, going for a walk or a run or playing sports or dancing does wonders for our mental and physical health.

This kind of modulated self-care, however, often does not take us into genuinely restful states that could be restorative. Making sure we attend the classes, thinking about how we look to others in the class, figuring out the best workout wardrobe, calculating the calories burned, or thinking about if we are doing the activity "right" just gives us more to do or to worry about.

During exercise, as we are walking or running or biking or hiking, our DMN thoughts may continue nonstop as we roll out prospective scenarios and review the recent past. In the gym, we might be watching TV or listening to music from our perch on the exercise bike or treadmill. Or we might walk with companions and be engaged in conversation. We are typically not paying much attention to our felt experiences.

These pervasive cultural practices keep us going and directed outward and away from the more prolonged and tender embrace of our restorative ESA. Modulated ESA is a solution but not a cure. It is a way of life that makes narrative, logical sense, but it has risks as well as benefits.

Restorative ESA is radically different. Feeling and sharing emotions and sensations more fully, with sufficient time to induce restorative ESA states, have additional long-term health benefits beyond those of simply talking about emotions or engaging in a yoga class or getting exercise. Opening up our emotions with others yields a sense of relief and inner peace. With repeated experiences of communicating with others what we are feeling, it becomes easier over time to tolerate negative emotions and both emotional and physical pain. Restorative practices help us let go of trying so hard to strategically modulate ourselves, and escape our out-of-control dysregulated thoughts and pains.

Unfortunately, restorative ESA does not always happen in therapy or classes meant to develop body awareness. Most forms of ESA practice are focused and task-oriented. There are postures and movements and routines to follow. There are discipline and rigor and the need to pay attention. There are talking and understanding and explaining by the leader or teacher about what we are doing and why. These activities are primarily about acquiring tools for self-modulation.

In my teaching and clinical practice, in my correspondence with readers of my writings, in discussions with practitioners of different therapeutic modalities that claim to promote ESA, and in everyday life, I find that the language of modulation is everywhere while the language of restoration is either not used or is not made salient.

Recovery from trauma, healing from illness, and the goals of most forms of psychotherapy and medical practices are all focused on regaining homeostasis (modulation) of thoughts, feelings, and functional body systems (cardiovascular, respiratory, digestive, urinary, and immune) and on getting back to being reasonably healthy and productive.

Modulation, without question, is central to well-being and to becoming reasonably happy and able to contribute to family and society. It is the primary route out of dysregulated ESA. If you start in a state of dysregulation, then gaining the ability to self-modulate is a necessary step toward personal growth. If some crucial parts of ourselves feel as if they have been broken, we now have these amazing modulatory practices like psychotherapy, yoga, and mindfulness meditation that get us back into a state of healthy productivity and well-being.

But there is more to life and well-being than modulation. With restorative ESA, there is Healing with a capital H, there is being fully alive in states of being without having to "do" or fix anything, and there is a profound sense of peace and rest that is fundamentally renewing. There are many books and practice modalities that teach about how to self-modulate. Although this book talks about modulation because it is one of the three states of ESA, modulation is not the main theme.

This book is instead about how to find restoration in everyday life. You can find books written by spiritual teachers and guides that also describe what I am calling restorative states of ESA. This book, however, is based in scientifically and clinically grounded evidence that hopefully speaks to both the thinking and feeling parts of ourselves.

Activities like taking a swim in the ocean or a hike in the wilderness to exercise, to achieve a personal fitness goal, or to be with someone on an adventure fall into the realm of modulated functioning. That kind of activity is fundamentally different from the restorative process of finding stillness and being completely overwhelmed and awed by the power of the sea or the intricate web of life in a wild forest. Modulation is a great fix for lots of things, but restoration is transformative.

The Neurophysiology of Felt Experience

This section is devoted to a more detailed explanation about the anatomy and physiology of the brain and the other body organs and tissues that support the ability to sense our inner condition via the three states of our embodied self-awareness. Like the discussions of the neural networks supporting TPN and DMN thinking in chapter 1, this section is here for readers who want to hear about the scientific research and understand better the highly attuned neurophysiological networks that are specifically dedicated to felt experience.

Let's begin with some review. In chapter 1, we saw that the neurophysiology of thought is separated into two different neural networks: the task-positive network (TPN) and the default-mode network (DMN). We also learned that these networks are mutually exclusive. When we are mind-wandering and reviewing our day in our DMN, we cannot at the same time be focused on a task or problem, and vice versa. The same is true for felt experience. We can be feeling something or we can be thinking about something, but not both at the same time.

Recall that felt experience is composed of interoceptive, proprioceptive, autonomic, and emotional feelings (see Table 1.2, p. 11). Each of these will be discussed in separate sections here. All forms of felt experience are supported by a complex cellular network that extends across multiple areas of the brain, the peripheral nervous system (see Figure 1.1, p. 3), the blood (Figure 1.2, p. 5), and other organic systems of the body.

All the neural networks for felt experience converge on the insula (see Figures 2.1–2.3 and 2.5), a region in the middle layer of the brain under the temporal lobe, which coalesces the bodily inputs for felt experience into awareness. The same neural pathways that send information to the insula to be transformed into our conscious awareness of felt experience also send information back into the sensorimotor and vital organ systems in order to help maintain homeostasis (balance, health) throughout the body.[4] Feeling ourselves is an essential component of maintaining health and balance in our body systems. Felt experience is

> the sense of the physiological condition of the entire body and of different bodily signals with the ... insula as a relevant brain site for the integration of homeostatic states of different bodily tissues with motivational and emotional processes, supporting feeling states and giving rise to conscious visceral perception.[5]

The prefrontal cortex is the part of the brain that regulates and organizes all the main functions of thought and feeling. Recall that the dorsomedial prefrontal cortex is the regulatory center for DMN thinking, while the dorsolateral prefrontal cortex is the site in the brain where focused attention is regulated in the TPN (see Figures 1.3, p. 15, and 1.5, p. 21). For felt experience, the regulatory center is the ventromedial (toward the eyes and in the middle layer) prefrontal cortex (Figures 2.1–2.3 and 2.5).*

The ventromedial prefrontal cortex works together with the insula to help maintain all these forms of felt experience in awareness for a sustained period of time. When the ventromedial prefrontal cortex is activated, we are more likely to be able to stay with felt experience and arrive at a state of restorative ESA.

As mentioned briefly at the end of the previous chapter, stress and trauma impair our ability to access felt experience. What happens in the brain is that the amygdala shuts down the ventromedial prefrontal cortex so that the feelings generated by the insula become impaired or distorted in our conscious awareness. This is analogous to how the amygdala can shut down the regulatory effects of the dorsomedial prefrontal cortex, thus shifting more-expansive DMN thinking into ruminative and dysregulated DMN thought.

When the amygdala blocks access to the regulating effects of the ventromedial prefrontal cortex, the resulting impairment of felt experience shows up in two basic ways. During the state of modulated ESA, we have only brief or no access to felt experience. The deactivation of the ventromedial prefrontal cortex suppresses our conscious awareness of felt experience.[6] The other form of impairment, which occurs primarily in dysregulated ESA, is that negative felt experiences—painful, anxious, or depressed feelings—become amplified and intense in such a way that we cannot modulate them.

The amygdala, while altering felt experience, also activates the hypothalamus to prepare the body to respond to the stressor. It does this in part by promoting the secretion of stress hormones into the blood and by creating a state of alertness and defensiveness via the autonomic nervous system (ANS; see Figure 2.4 and discussion of autonomic feelings to follow).

---

* Recall from chapter 1 that another part of the medial prefrontal cortex, the dorsomedial prefrontal cortex, works with the posterior cingulate cortex to organize coherent imaginative off-task DMN thoughts about ourselves and our social relationships. The dorsal portion of the medial prefrontal cortex is located toward the top of the head; the ventral portion is located toward the bottom of the head.

This complex network (insula, prefrontal cortex, amygdala, hypothalamus) is the brain's center for shifting our bodies between restorative, modulated, and dysregulated ESA states. Therapies and education programs that enhance access to felt experience and to states of modulated and restorative ESA are actually rewiring this part of the nervous system in order to dampen amygdala activity and strengthen the availability of the ventromedial prefrontal cortex to regulate and expand felt experience.[7] (This shifting between states—in particular the shift from a dysregulated to a modulated state and from modulated to restorative—is discussed further in chapter 4.)

Interoceptive Feelings

Interoceptive feelings are those connected with body sensations such as pain/ease, warm/cold, illness/health, itchy, dizzy, thirsty, tingling and chills, numb, tense, flushed, or strong/weak. These feelings begin in the sensory-interoceptive receptors at the nerve endings of very long peripheral nerve cells that connect different parts of the body with the spinal cord and, from there, to the brain stem.*

Muscles, for example, have multiple types of receptors, such as for stretch and for fatigue. Receptors in the skin sense movement at the base of a hair follicle and pressure (these are usually connected to the interoceptive experience of different types of touch). There are also receptors in the skin for vibration, heat and cold, and pain. Recall from chapter 1 that, unlike the blood that reaches every cell in the body, peripheral nerve cells do not connect to every cell. Each receptor in skeletal muscle tissue, for example, is connected to what is called a *motor unit*, a clump of adjacent muscle cells.[8]

---

* Nerve cells have a central nucleus from which extend appendages called *axons* and *dendrites*. These appendages transmit chemical (neurotransmitter) and electrical messages from one nerve cell to another via connectors called *synapses*. In peripheral nerve cells, the distance between the receptor at the nerve ending and the spinal cord where that cell makes its first synapse could be as long as one or two feet, or half a meter.

The electrical and chemical signals from the interoceptive sensory receptors throughout the body travel along their connected peripheral nerve cells. Peripheral nerve cells are sometimes called *fibers* because each cell can run along an entire arm or a leg, very thin and long, before connecting into the spinal cord. Interoceptive peripheral nerve cells connect specifically to a pathway at the dorsal (back) side of the spinal cord, into so-called Aδ (pronounced "A-delta") and C spinal cord nerve fibers. The interoceptive peripheral nerves and the spinal Aδ and C fibers *do not* have a protective coating called *myelin*.

Myelin is like the plastic or rubber insulation around a copper electrical wire. This insulation prevents our getting shocked if we touch the wire, and it also ensures that the electricity moving along the wire stays contained within the wire. The lack of myelin makes the neural transmission of chemical and electrical interoceptive information between body and brain a bit of a leaky system. Much like an uninsulated electrical wire will leak electricity, an unmyelinated nerve cell will also leak its electrical and chemical neurotransmitters as they move through the body (more on this leaky property of interoception soon).

These spinal interoceptive fibers ultimately connect into the brain stem's periaqueductal gray area, and from there into the thalamus (located in the very center of the brain), and finally into the insula (in the middle layer of the brain) where felt experience is brought into conscious awareness.[9] The thalamus (Figure 2.1) keeps track of the body locations of the interoceptive signals before it relays those signals to the insula.

This function of the thalamus to "remember" the body location of interoceptive signals helps explain why our body awareness is felt not in the head where our thoughts seem to be located, but rather at specific locations within the body. An itch is felt at a site on the skin where there might be a rash or bug bite. A sore muscle feels sore at the site of that particular hurt muscle.

This is another reason why the mind-body dichotomy, discussed in chapter 1, is not helpful. Even though thought seems to come from the brain or the head, and even though an ache seems to come from a specific location in the body, both thought and felt experience are created in conscious awareness via complex neural connections that extend throughout the body and brain.

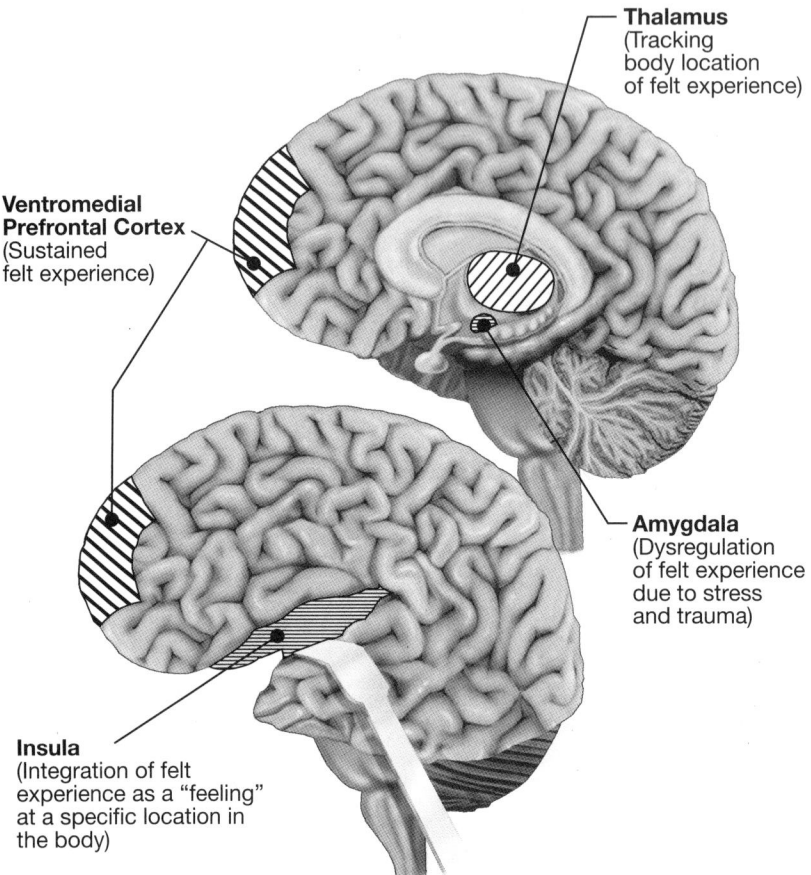

FIGURE 2.1: *Neural network for interoception.*

Proprioceptive Feelings

Proprioceptive feelings tell us about how different parts of the body are moving in relation to other parts, and they help us with motor coordination and skilled movements, balance, sense of boundaries, and our personal experience of our body size and shape. These proprioceptive feelings arise from the same interoceptive stretch and fatigue receptors in the muscles, in similar receptors in the tendons that connect muscle to bone, and in the orientation and balance receptors in the ear canals.

Proprioceptive feelings also come into our awareness via the insula. Like interoceptive feelings, proprioceptive feelings travel through the thalamus, which tracks body locations. Before arriving at the insula, however, proprioceptive feelings are routed through the posterior parietal cortex and sensorimotor cortices in the exterior (neocortex) lobes of the brain (Figure 2.2).* Like interoception, proprioception is experienced at particular locations around the body.

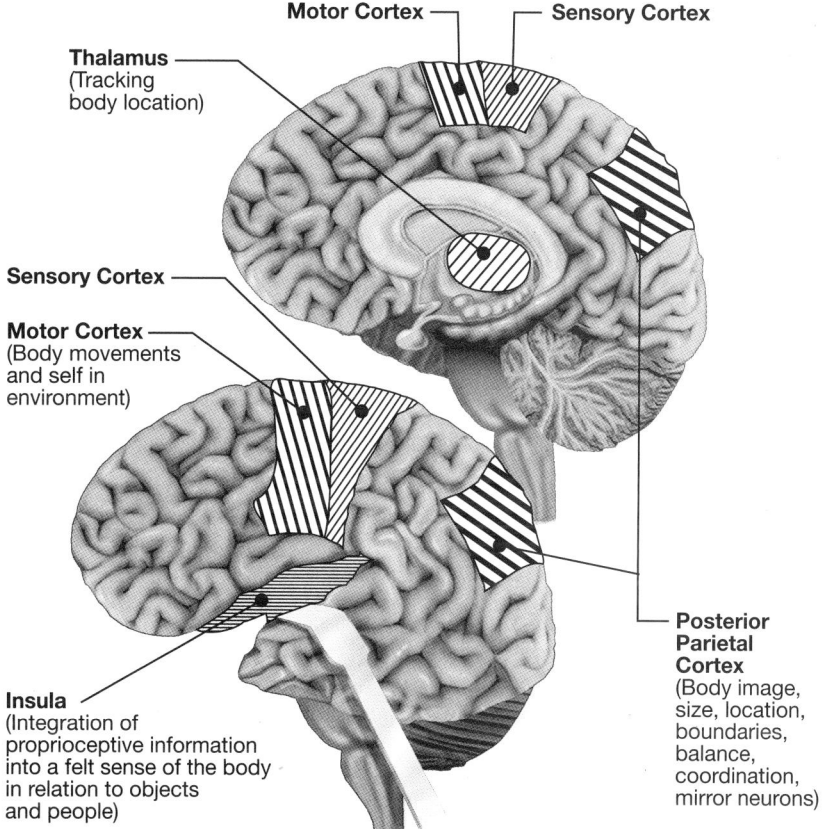

FIGURE 2.2: *Neural network for proprioception.*

---

* Proprioception involves the posterior *parietal* cortex located in the parietal lobe of the outer layer of the brain (Figure 2.2). Note that this is different from the posterior *cingulate* cortex—located in the middle layer of the brain—that generates self-related DMN thinking (see Figure 1.5, p. 21).

In the case of proprioception, however, the body location information is "saved" in the sensorimotor cortex; the posterior parietal cortex puts all this information into a schema or map of the whole body. The posterior parietal cortex contains not only the brain centers for creating this map of information coming from inside the body, but also information about the body via exteroception from outside the body. The map in the posterior parietal cortex, therefore, helps us organize and coordinate our movements within our own body and also in relationship to the environment and with other people.

The posterior parietal cortex is also one of the few locations in the brain that contain so-called mirror neurons, those that allow us to notice and follow the movements of other people, to imitate, to empathize by watching others' emotional expressions in their face and whole body, and to identify our own image in a mirror.[10] This mutual coordination of movements and postures happens naturally when people are walking together, playing sports together, dancing, making love, or anything that requires between-person embodied coordination.

Proprioception includes the feeling of whether or not all these complex co-occurring movements—both within our own body and those movements we make with other people—are comfortable and coordinated. As with interoceptors, proprioceptors—from the muscles, tendons, and ear canal—connect via similar nonmyelinated peripheral nerves through the dorsal spinal cord and eventually into the posterior parietal cortex, the sensorimotor cortex, and, like all felt experience, the insula (Figure 2.2).

Spontaneous movements like yawning often occur with stretching the muscles around the mouth and jaw and may be accompanied by shaking the head and stretching the arms and legs, thus activating proprioceptors.[11] Twitching and body spasms also activate the stretch receptors and, like yawning, give us the felt sense of the boundaries and extensions of the body within itself and into the environment.[12] We can only stretch our muscles so far before it becomes painful.

The proprioceptors in the ear give us a sense of balance and stability but also contribute in important ways to our sense of self in the body. Middle-ear proprioception, in particular, provides the felt experience of moving through space, the boundaries of our bodies, our body image relating to our sense of our shape and size, our sense that we are living in this body and not another one, and our location in relation to other bodies and objects. We can feel the boundaries of our skin, what is inside of us vs. outside.[13]

Proprioception via the mirror neurons in the posterior parietal cortex and seeing our own mirror image can create the sense of whether we feel fat or thin, short or tall, and create an impression about how other people may judge our appearance.[14] In chapter 1, we saw that felt experience can become impaired under conditions of stress and trauma, and in this chapter we named that as dysregulated ESA. Proprioception can also become impaired when we are in dysregulated ESA.

If our proprioception is dysregulated, we might feel fat even though we are of average weight, which might predispose us to an eating disorder. We might feel dissatisfied with our body shape or appearance even though other people may see us differently than we see ourselves. When proprioception is dysregulated, we quickly move from the felt sense of our body shape, size, and movement into self-deprecating DMN ruminative judgments about how we look to ourselves and to other people (more on dysregulated body image and eating disorders in chapter 5). Or we might have porous interpersonal boundaries and let others get too close in a way that is ultimately harmful.

Even if our body shape is more or less in the average range, we might have thoughts that our breasts are too large or small, too flat or pointy, that our face or hair or eyes are unattractive. Dysregulated thinking and feeling about our body are relatively common as we compare ourselves to some "perfect" cultural ideal created by the many forms of media images and advertising in which we are immersed. Teens and young adults, whose bodies are growing and changing rapidly, are particularly susceptible to distortions of body image and the resulting dysregulated feelings, thoughts, and behaviors.

Alternatively, we can decide, using our TPN, that our body shape and size, our skin color, our hair, or our sexual identity is just as it should be. We can learn modulated ways of thinking about ourselves so that we feel comfortable living in this particular body. To the extent that our body image and ethnic or sexual identity give us pleasure in being exactly who we are, that we can feel ourselves just being ourselves without thought or worry, our body image can be a source of ongoing restorative comfort and peace.

Weronika Grantham, a faculty member at Józef Piłsudski University of Physical Education in Warsaw, Poland, writes about her restorative experience of dancing as a young child:

> In the moments of my spontaneous dance, I was not consciously reflecting upon my experience of dancing but was fully immersed in it. I also experienced moments of oneness—a unity, the lack of dualism between my body and mind. I felt as one, moving, flowing and expressing myself.[15]

At the age of twelve, around the time she was coming into puberty, Grantham was diagnosed with scoliosis, a curvature of the spine. At that point she began to experience dysregulated feelings and thoughts about not only the shape of her spine but the rest of her developing female body.

At age seventeen, still wanting to dance, she enrolled in a ballet school in Krakow, Poland, but the rigor and conformity of the school left her feeling worse about herself and her body. When she was twenty, she moved to Belgium to attend a school of modern dance where she discovered dance improvisation and yoga. These practices helped her to come back to herself:

> I was able to feel myself as a more embodied being and started to experience more moments of well-being. I began noticing once more that my body speaks the non-verbal language of feeling, sensation, and movement. Looking back now I know this was a turning point towards my healing.[16]

From there, she moved to the UK and completed a bachelor's degree in Dance and Movement Studies and Healing Arts at the University of Derby and then got a master's degree in Dance and Somatic Wellbeing: Connections to the Living Body at the University of Central Lancashire. She went on to become a somatic educator and eventually returned to her native Warsaw to study and teach about embodied awareness and movement. In addition to finding restoration in movement and dance, she also learned important skills of modulated proprioception:

> I was using my felt-sense, rather than just purely focusing on the visual appearance of the body. Via increased bodily awareness, I was able to distinguish between different levels of muscular tension

in different parts of my body. This allowed me to decide for myself whether I needed rest, or whether I needed active movement. I was actively responding to my body's needs. I knew how to take care of my body a bit better.[17]

ENHANCED PROPRIOCEPTION FOLLOWING LOSS

Most often, proprioception operates in the background of our awareness. We "know" we "have" a body, that our body has parts and appendages, that it moves in certain ways. One way that the felt experience of proprioception comes into our embodied self-awareness is when we are learning new skills. Riding a bike, learning a sport, or doing tai chi requires us to pay attention in the present moment to our sense of balance and coordination.

Of course, we are using our balance every time we walk or stand, every time we run or jump. For a baby or child first learning these motor skills, balance proprioception becomes salient in ESA, but once we've got these abilities they become second nature, meaning that we don't have to think about them and we don't have to even directly feel them.

Another way in which proprioception becomes a salient felt experience is after some kind of loss of ability, or loss of a body part. An independent embodied movement practitioner and scholar living in London, Fiona O'Neill, has written about the felt experience of having a mastectomy.[18] After recovery from the surgery, she put on a bra with a foam prosthetic breast. She was immediately struck by the feel of her upper arm brushing against this prosthesis.

This experience made her aware of her changed body shape due to the breast removal, but more importantly for her, she realized that she had felt this sensation many times before with her natural breasts. It's just that she never really paid attention to this feeling. The loss of her breast somehow enhanced her proprioceptive awareness.

In the same article, O'Neill describes the experience of people with hearing aids. With their hearing restored after years of hearing loss, people may suddenly become aware of sounds that their bodies make in relation to things, like the sound of their arm moving in a shirt sleeve, or the 3D orientation to the world around them that locates their body in space via sound (rather than vision).

As a hearing-impaired person, I have a similar experience whenever I take out or put in my hearing aids. Taking them out, the loss of sonic cues that orient me in the world and tune me in to my family members is always a bit startling. I feel more vulnerable and lost, and my anxiety level may rise. When I put the hearing aids on in the morning, I am also startled in the opposite way: there is a whole soundscape in the house I was not attuned to. When that rushes in as I turn on the hearing aids, it suddenly places me "here" in relation to sounds coming from other rooms or from outside the house.

In another personal example, my vision some years ago had become cloudy and gray due to cataracts. I had gotten used to this diminished visual sense until it began to impair my ability to navigate in the world. After I received cataract surgery to replace the lenses in both eyes with prosthetic lenses, I was shocked into a new awareness of color and the clarity of space. My new lenses also corrected a lifelong visual impairment of extreme nearsightedness, so there was the additional shock of seeing clearly at a distance without glasses or contacts, as if there was no longer a boundary between me and the world.

The point of all these examples is that after a loss of a body part or sensory modality, a partial or full repair or replacement can bring us into our body in ways that we had somehow forgotten. A similar effect happens when we change residences or travel. Having gotten used to location and orientation to our surroundings at home, they fade into the background, no longer salient in felt experience. In a new place, we become once again attuned to ordinary proprioceptive felt experiences about space, boundaries, and our location and orientation in the world.

Autonomic Feelings

Autonomic feelings are another form of felt experiences, those that come from the organic functions of the body—the functions that keep us alive. Cardiovascular autonomic feelings may include sensing our heart racing or slowing, or feeling the pulsations of the blood in different parts of the body. Respiratory autonomic feelings include the sense that breathing is easy or difficult, free and natural or constricted in some way, such as having congestion in the lungs.

Digestive autonomic feelings are those of fullness or hunger, ease or bloating, gastric distress, and bowel movements. Urinary and genital autonomic feelings include bladder fullness or emptiness and sexual arousal or disinterest. Because autonomic feelings are composed of the pulsations and movements that keep us alive, some people claim that they are at the core of what it means to have a sense of aliveness in a human body.[19]

Like the other forms of felt experience discussed earlier, autonomic feelings also arise from receptors at the ends of long peripheral nerve fibers. These receptors are located in the muscle cells of the internal organs, so-called smooth muscles. These are the muscles that open and close the pupils of the eyes depending on lighting conditions, create heartbeats in coronary muscles, move blood via contractions of the muscles in our arteries and veins, move food and waste through our digestive system, and control movements in the urinary, reproductive, and genital-sexual systems.

Smooth muscles contract and relax rhythmically across the entire muscular structure. The tubular-shaped smooth muscles of the intestines and blood vessels, for example, move in a wavelike motion that pushes the food or blood in a single direction along the pathways of these organs. The heart moves in a wave from bottom to top with each beat as blood is transported through the ventricles and out into the aorta to circulate around the body.

These smooth-muscle movements are involuntary, paced and controlled by a dedicated brain-body network called the *autonomic nervous system* (ANS). Most of the time, because the muscle movements inspired by the ANS are involuntary and automatic, we don't really notice all the throbbing, beating, moving, stirring, and flowing that supports being alive. But if we allow ourselves to pay attention, we can notice that our ANS and its accompanying autonomic felt experience are equipped to continually remind us that we are indeed a living, pulsing being.

Whereas autonomic receptors connect to the smooth muscles, interoceptive and proprioceptive receptors and their peripheral nerves are connected to our *skeletal muscles*, those that attach to a bone via a tendon at the end of the muscle (hence, skeletal). Usually, the muscle spans a moving joint where bones meet. Unlike smooth muscles, skeletal muscles are voluntary—but they can still be responsible for autonomic feelings.

In addition to the interoceptive nerves that sense stretch and fatigue and are connected to each motor unit in the skeletal muscles, there are also motor nerves from each motor unit. These motor nerves connect into a dedicated pathway in the spinal cord that is closest to the front of the body (the ventral pathway, different from the dorsal pathway of the interoceptive nerves) and then into the sensorimotor cortex of the brain that sends signals for a skeletal muscle to contract or relax.

All the cells in a single motor unit move together to create either low-level isometric contractions (and also chronic muscle tension) or high-level muscle contractions that move bones across a joint.* The motor-control nerves from the cell body and those in the ventral spinal cord are, unlike the interoceptive nerves, covered with a protective sheath of myelin. This myelin coating increases the speed and fidelity of transmission along the peripheral nerves and in the spinal cord, allowing for precise and fine-tuned movements such as those involved in writing, drawing, playing a musical instrument, speaking, dancing, or doing athletics.

So, some autonomic feelings arise in the stretch and fatigue receptors of the smooth muscles of the internal organs as they expand and contract involuntarily. When the smooth muscles in the digestive system are overly

---

* A few skeletal muscles do not move bones across a joint. The tiny muscles behind the eyes, for example, attach to skull bones at one end and to the back of the eyeball at the other. These muscles allow you to move your eyes left or right, up or down. These eye muscles, like all skeletal muscles and their motor nerves, are for voluntary movements.

expanded for a prolonged period, we can feel gassy or constipated or that we ate too much. When they are overly contracted, we can feel nausea or reflux or pain.

We saw in a previous section that not all interoceptive feelings come from the skeletal muscles; there are receptors in the skin, hair follicles, nose, ears, and eyes. Similarly, not all autonomic feelings arise in the smooth muscles. Autonomic feelings also can be evoked by hormones released into the bloodstream as part of the activity of the hypothalamus, which is part of the ANS (see Figure 1.2, p. 5). Hormonal autonomic feelings can include energy (feeling aroused or "up") or fatigue (feeling low, tired, down), interpersonal warmth and closeness, feelings of stress and tension, sexual feelings including attraction or repulsion, or orgasm and release, and all the complex body feelings of menstruation, pregnancy, childbirth, nursing, and menopause (which can occur as a result of aging-related hormonal changes in all gender types, not only in cisgender women). As shown in Figure 2.3, both smooth-muscle and hormonal autonomic feelings are processed in the deep or limbic areas of the brain, including the hypothalamus and pituitary, amygdala, brain stem periaqueductal gray area, and finally the insula.[20]

The ANS keeps the heart beating, the lungs breathing, and vital hormones flowing, thus maintaining our aliveness. It also has another function: the detection of safety vs. threat or challenge. This means that the ANS regulates changes in the action of smooth muscles and hormones throughout the whole body in response to how the nervous system perceives safety or danger.

A sense of danger or safety can come from either the environment outside the body (a threating situation vs. a situation in which we feel protected) or within the body itself (emotional or physical pain, or body memories of prior trauma, or an illness or dysfunction in one of the organ systems composed of smooth muscles vs. a sense of inner calm, peace, or absence of pain). Depending upon whether the ANS senses danger or safety, these smooth muscles can contract or relax to widen or narrow our field of vision and hearing, increase or decrease our heart rate, open or narrow our blood vessels, expand or constrict respiration, activate or slow digestion and urination, or create genital erections or flaccidity (see Figure 2.4).

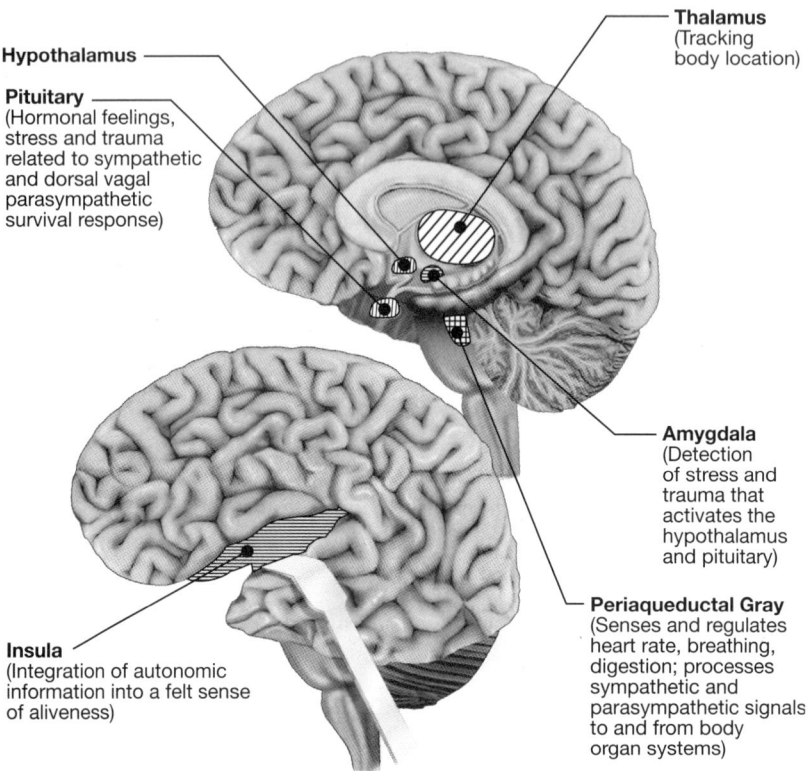

Thalamus
(Tracking
body location)

Hypothalamus ⎯⎯⎯⎯

Pituitary ⎯⎯⎯⎯
(Hormonal feelings,
stress and trauma
related to sympathetic
and dorsal vagal
parasympathetic
survival response)

Amygdala
(Detection
of stress and
trauma that
activates the
hypothalamus
and pituitary)

Periaqueductal Gray
(Senses and regulates
heart rate, breathing,
digestion; processes
sympathetic and
parasympathetic signals
to and from body
organ systems)

Insula
(Integration of autonomic
information into a felt sense
of aliveness)

FIGURE 2.3: *Neural network for autonomic feelings.*

The ANS accomplishes this body regulation in response to safety or challenge via its two main branches: sympathetic and parasympathetic. Activation of the sympathetic branch of the ANS during modulated ESA states is an adaptive and functional response to challenge: increased heart rate, preparation for action, muscle activation and tension, slowed digestion and urination, heightened vigilance and focused attention, and constricted respiration.

Sympathetic activation also supports being productive, using our TPN and DMN, and engaging with tasks in the world. Sympathetic activation typically triggers the adrenal glands to release the hormone cortisol, a blood

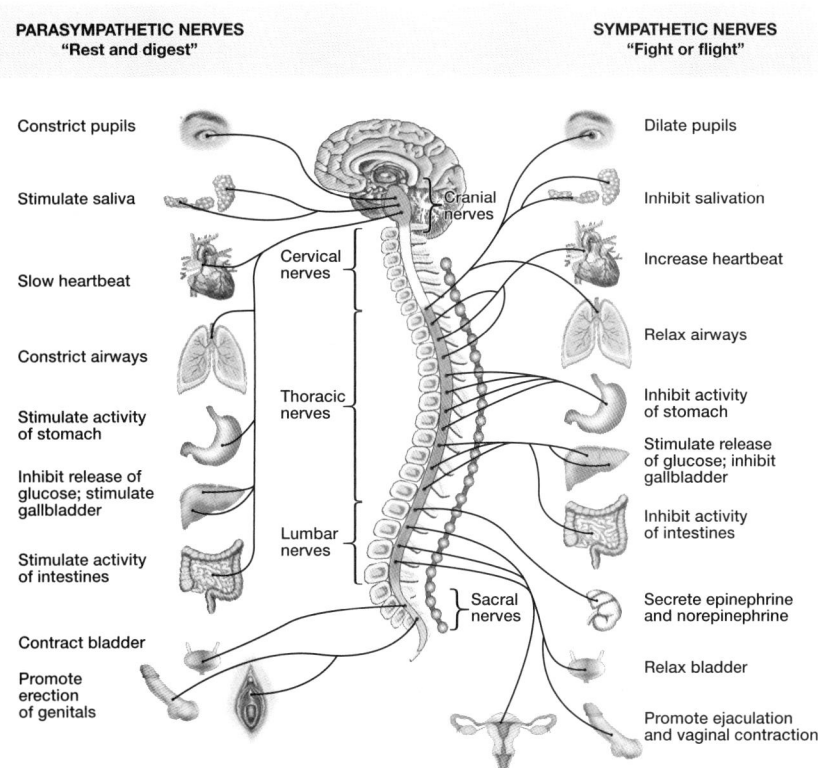

FIGURE 2.4: *The sympathetic and parasympathetic branches of the autonomic nervous system.*

sugar that helps power the body through the sympathetic activity. Any type of focused attention requires the metabolic energy of cortisol and the activation of the sympathetic branch of the ANS. We can be focused in our thoughts (such as TPN problem solving or DMN rumination) or focused on a motor activity (such as making music, dancing, athletics, or physical labor). This sympathetically supported focused attention can be on a specific part of the body or on our thoughts, or it can be a focus on the environment using exteroception. Sympathetic activation widens the pupils, increases heart rate, creates a state of alertness or vigilance, and prepares the body to direct attention to a specific activity (Figure 2.4).

The sympathetic ANS is also associated with dysregulated ESA. The amygdala and hypothalamus play a role in whether the body reacts to a challenge in a way that can be modulated, or whether that challenge may be experienced as dysregulated: overwhelming, threatening, or dangerous. In those circumstances, the sympathetic nervous system evokes the survival responses of fight or flight.

Fight is a general metaphor for any kind of defensive action related to self-protection. There might be actual fighting and self-defense when one is being attacked or assaulted. One can also use TPN and DMN thoughts and words to express anger or to justify and defend one's actions during a confrontation with another person. We can also fight with ourselves in states of dysregulated ESA, such as when we experience self-doubt, become angry with ourselves, or turn to self-harming actions (self-cutting, eating unhealthy foods, drinking too much alcohol, or indulging in substance abuse) as a way to fight off whatever may arise in us that feels unpleasant or unwanted.

Flight is a metaphor for the defensive act of running away from external or internal threats. During an assault, one can try to escape, run, or hide. During threatening social encounters, flight behaviors might include looking away, walking away, refusing to respond, or avoiding certain people or topics. We can also flee from our own felt experiences by active suppression or inhibition of our true feelings.

In fight or flight dysregulated states, we cannot easily turn off the high sympathetic arousal. Dysregulation is the feeling of being stuck or trapped. This means that we remain sympathetically aroused and continue to secrete cortisol even after the immediate danger has passed.

Chronic and dysregulated sympathetic arousal and elevated cortisol— from an ongoing threatening situation such as living with an abuser or in a war zone, or from a past or recent trauma—are unhealthy. They can slow immune system repair functions and increase inflammation.[21]

Sympathetic arousal that is "stuck on" can also make cortisol receptor sites in the amygdala and other brain regions hypersensitive. This means that even if we find ourselves out of danger and in a safer environment, a "normal" level of sympathetic activation that would otherwise be modulated and productive is sufficient to trigger in us a dysregulated state of fight or flight.[22]

Activation of the parasympathetic branch of the ANS allows us to "rest and digest," slow down, and breathe easier; it supports healthy function of most of our body systems. With the accompanying release of the hormone oxytocin, parasympathetic activation also provides feelings of warmth and connection, well-being, peace, and contentment.

Parasympathetic activation supports sexual arousal by opening genital blood vessels and increasing blood flow to support erectile function in the penis and clitoris during situations of closeness and shared mutual pleasure. The increased blood flow also enhances sensitivity to touch via the skin. As shown in Figure 2.4, these functions, plus bladder release that supports ease of urination, arise in the sacral portion of the spinal cord rather than from the brain stem.

Also from Figure 2.4, you can see that the sympathetic nerves branch off from nerve roots in the spinal cord and into different body organs. The main nerve of the parasympathetic branch of the ANS—the vagus nerve—on the other hand, has its roots in the brain stem periaqueductal gray area (see Figure 2.3). The vagus nerve has two main branches (not shown in Figure 2.4). One arises from the ventral part of the periaqueductal gray (toward the front of the upper neck) and the other from the dorsal region of the periaqueductal gray (toward the back of the upper neck).

The ventral vagal system allows us to find moments of felt experience during modulated states and to make eye contact and engage with others in modulated and supportive social connections. Dorsal vagal activation, when we feel safe, is one of the main contributors to restorative states of ESA. Dorsal vagal activation during safety promotes what has been called *immobilization without fear.* It creates the possibility of feeling oneness or closeness with another person, both physically and emotionally, without a need to think about or do anything. This is a restorative state that does not need words or explanations or trying or performing.[23]

We might be resting in someone's arms, being held, holding hands while sitting together, or just being in the same place together and feeling the shared connection. It might be a parent holding a child, or romantic partners, or close friends who feel safe enough with each other to "just be" together and feel the presence, warmth, contact, or sense of love, affection, and closeness.

In addition to dorsal vagal immobilization without fear that contributes to restorative states, the dorsal branch of the vagus nerve is also activated during dysregulated states of threat and danger. When we feel safe, the dorsal vagal system slows us down and induces feelings of quiet and deep rest. When we sense danger, the dorsal vagal system also slows us down to the point of not being able to move or respond—by fight or flight—to the danger. *Dorsal vagal immobilization with fear* is a self-protective response metaphorically called *freeze.*

When we cannot actively defend ourselves with fight or flight actions, our ANS turns on this freeze response. Freezing occurs when we are suddenly confronted with a situation that we have no capacity to handle or process. Freeze is a common response to a sexual, physical, or even verbal assault. It can happen during an impending automobile accident when we find ourselves unable to respond. Our mind goes blank or our thoughts may be racing, but we can't move or do anything. Whatever is happening is somehow beyond comprehension and creates a state of shock, paralysis, or immobility.

Freeze is a potential means of survival during an assault because it may seem to the attackers that we are unconscious or lifeless and there is nothing else for them to accomplish. It evolved across many animal species over millions of years because when prey animals can't fight or escape, freezing makes their bodies go limp. Many predator animals lose interest in their prey under such conditions and simply walk away.

In most human situations, the inability to respond can create lifelong states of trauma because after the assault we are left with dysregulated ruminative DMN thoughts about why we could not escape or fight back. We keep asking ourselves why we could not avoid an automobile accident when our body become frozen, or we become stuck in self-blame when our immobilization could not prevent ourselves or someone close to us from becoming harmed.

The "what ifs" keep replaying in ruminative DMN thoughts along with feelings of shame and helplessness. Many forms of therapy for treating such trauma states rely on helping people monitor their dysregulated thought patterns and develop more productive and helpful thoughts. The objective truth is that there was nothing we could do because our ANS survival strategies took over—we literally had no voluntary control over our actions. Embodied therapies can help people feel the frozen state and then feel themselves regaining their felt experiences and self-modulatory abilities.

We'll finish this section on autonomic feelings with the observation that the broad or open type of attention that is most conducive to entering states of restorative ESA is, in fact, a parasympathetic state. We have more access to this kind of free-floating attention when we feel safe enough to let go of any kind of focus and just let ourselves be taken and transformed in the present moment.

Emotional Feelings

As shown in Figure 2.5, emotional feelings are formed in the insula, amygdala, anterior cingulate cortex,* orbitofrontal cortex, and supplementary motor area, which links to the sensorimotor cortex for the creation of the muscle movements of emotion expressions in the face and body.[24] Like all felt experience, emotion is brought into awareness via the insula.[25] Like each of the other forms of felt experience reviewed in this section, the insula connects to unique parts of the nervous system, giving each form (interoception, proprioception, autonomic feeling, and emotion) its particular experiential quality.

Emotions are *embodied values* that are added to each of the other forms of felt experiences. Embodied values are different from values that come from judgments in thought. Emotional values are the felt sense that interoceptive, proprioceptive, and autonomic feelings are "liked" or "disliked," "pleasurable" or "painful," or the sense that we want "more" or "less," or that we want to "approach" or "avoid."

The orbitofrontal cortex creates the sense of emotional value, while the anterior cingulate cortex initiates (via its links to the sensorimotor circuits) the movements and expressions related to that value. The value of "like" or "good" goes with movements related to approach and positive emotional expressions. The value of "dislike" or "bad" creates movements related to avoidance and negative emotional expressions.

---

* Note the difference between the *posterior* cingulate cortex—located in the middle layer of the brain—which generates self-related DMN thinking (see Figure 1.5, p. 21), and the *anterior* cingulate cortex, which is part of the network that forms self-related emotional experiences.

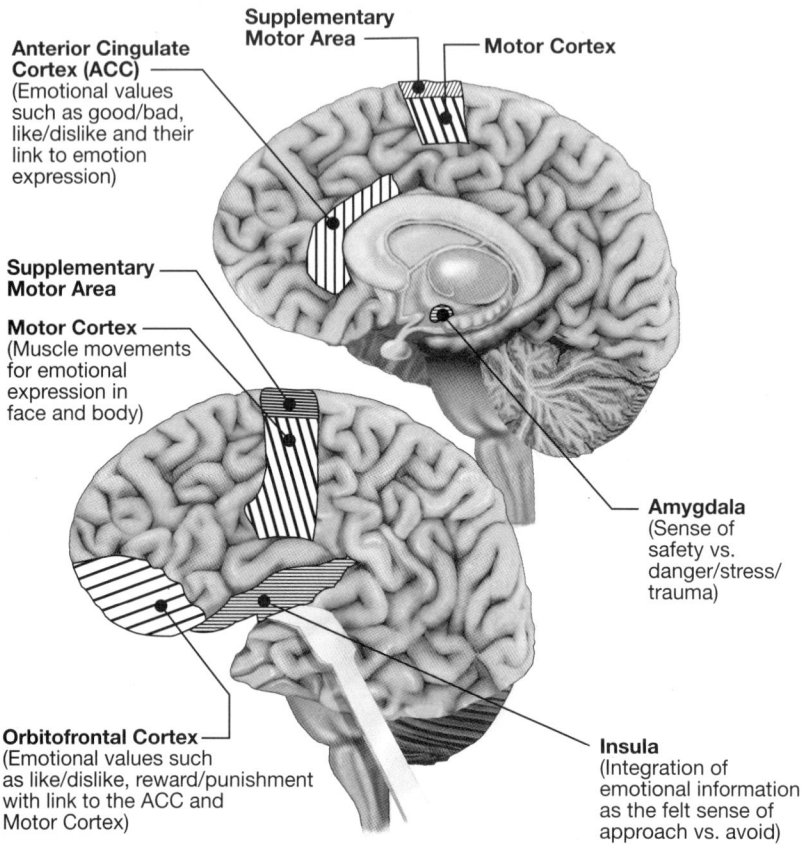

Supplementary Motor Area

Motor Cortex

Anterior Cingulate Cortex (ACC)
(Emotional values such as good/bad, like/dislike and their link to emotion expression)

Supplementary Motor Area

Motor Cortex
(Muscle movements for emotional expression in face and body)

Amygdala
(Sense of safety vs. danger/stress/ trauma)

Orbitofrontal Cortex
(Emotional values such as like/dislike, reward/punishment with link to the ACC and Motor Cortex)

Insula
(Integration of emotional information as the felt sense of approach vs. avoid)

FIGURE 2.5: *Neural network for emotion.*

Consider the emotion of disgust, which typically creates the feeling of wanting to avoid a particularly unpleasant odor, or image, or person. We may also have feelings of disgust toward our own body: toward an interoception of being uncomfortably warm, or a proprioception of dislike of our body shape or size, or an autonomic feeling of digestive upset.

Disgust may evoke interoceptive feelings such as "crawling" skin, a burning feeling in the nose or throat, or a feeling of nausea or wanting to gag. Proprioceptive feelings such as movements away from the noxious situation can also accompany disgust, while there is likely to be sympathetic activation to impel strategies to escape. The emotion of disgust is the body's evaluation (repulsiveness) of all those interoceptive, proprioceptive, and autonomic feelings.

Conversely, we can feel emotionally attracted to different smells, sights, and individuals. That emotional evaluation of attraction co-occurs with interoceptive feelings like warmth, softness, and vulnerability. Generally speaking, people high in interoceptive awareness are more likely to be able to feel their emotional states.[26] Proprioceptive feelings might lead to more physical closeness and movements like touching or hugging. Autonomically, we may have erotic feelings or a sense of relaxation that comes from being close to someone or something that we love.

Emotional feelings, in other words, are the ways in which we form a relationship to all the other felt experiences.[27] Having a relationship to our felt experiences means that for each one, we have some kind of emotional push or pull. In general, therefore, all the forms of felt experience are imbued with emotional values. Emotion is so important that chapter 6 is devoted entirely to this topic.

Experiential Exercise: Fuzzy Feelings

As mentioned earlier in this chapter, the peripheral nerves of felt experience that connect a particular body region to the spinal cord, as well as the spinal conduction fibers, are not myelinated. As a consequence, the Aδ (A-delta) and C neural pathways in the dorsal spinal cord that link the periphery to the brain are more "leaky" and conduct more slowly than the motor-control pathways. The felt experiences that coalesce in the insula, therefore, are not as high fidelity as the conduction of motor-nerve movement information into the sensorimotor cortex.

The slow conduction speeds and the resulting "fuzziness" of the information that reaches the brain explain why the act of discerning our felt experience is often slow and why it takes a while for us to find and feel its source within the body. This also explains why, in order to fully feel an ache or pulsation or temperature or pressure in a way that brings restorative relief, we have to stop all doing and thinking and settle into a place of quiet listening using a free-floating or diffuse kind of attention.

You could try as hard as you can to localize, define, and contain felt experience using your power of focused attention from the dorsolateral prefrontal cortex and TPN network. Basically, you'd be wasting your energy. No amount of concerted effort will bring something into focus that is inherently out of focus. Getting closer to our fuzzy feelings is going to take practice in not-focusing and not-doing.

This same fuzzy neural conduction mechanism helps explain what has been called *referred pain*—the pain felt in one area of the body (such as a headache) has its origin in another area (such as neck and shoulder muscles or the gut). Symptoms of a heart attack, for example, can show up as nausea or stomach pain, shooting pains in the arms, jaw pain, or lightheadedness in addition to chest tightness. The leaky conduction pathways allow inputs from one organ, one muscle, or a segment of skin tissue to jump over to a different C-fiber pathway in the dorsal spinal cord. When those signals arrive in the thalamus, they are "labeled" as coming from the referred location before being sent on to the insula.[28]

For all these reasons, the harder you try to focus on and pin down any kind of felt experience, the more slippery it becomes. The lack of myelination of the felt-experience nerve pathways means that body sensations are more like a watercolor than an oil painting, more like slightly out-of-focus photos compared to sharp images. They are elusive, and their precise origin is not completely determined or clear. We need to give ourselves lots of time and practice in order to allow a felt experience to "emerge" as a reasonably well-formed entity in our awareness.

For this exercise, settle into a safe and quiet place and notice which aches or pains call to you. In order to better locate the source, it may help to apply touch pressure to the general area of your body that feels discomfort, either by yourself or with someone else helping you, until you isolate the particular place that is hurting. Maybe the pain is in a superficial or deep muscle? Maybe it is coming from a joint or internal organ? Maybe you have an insect bite or a rash on the surface of your skin?

Because of the fuzziness of any single peripheral nerve and its spinal pathway, adding another source of felt experiences—like touch—to whatever arrives in the insula from tissues around the area of the pain helps more clearly locate its origin. Compared to the hare-paced rapid and instantaneous generation of ideas and thoughts in the TPN or DMN, or the execution of skilled motor movements, felt experience is a tortoise. It takes slowing down, practice, repetition, education, and support to find our feelings. But there is typically a big payoff that comes from taking all the time we need— remember who won the race!

Letting your attention be broad, you are more likely to feel into multiple locations around that area of the body without any effort or direction. Allowing your attention to be called to this broader complex of feelings is similar to the example just given, of tactile poking around an affected area until you more clearly discover the source of the problem. If you want to approach any kind of ache or discomfort in a restorative way, your broad-based attention may, in fact, lead you to other aspects of felt experience that are possibly connected in some way to the ache.

Perhaps you might suddenly remember that the ache began during an argument, or as the result of an accident, an overuse injury, a prior trauma, or a latent health condition that had been dormant. You might have memories (something hit you or you smashed into something, part of proprioceptive felt experience). You might have emotions that come up around the ache such as frustration or shame for letting this happen, or discouragement that your "old" condition may be returning.

Having a restorative ESA experience of this ache means that you open up to and allow all of these feelings to emerge in your awareness. It means that you just let them happen and feel them instead of resisting the feelings (fight), ignoring what is coming up (flight), or using modulated thinking to get yourself out of the challenging feeling.

This may surprise you, but if you can stay in the present moment for a sufficiently long period of time, and if you permit all your felt experiences to arise spontaneously, *you will almost certainly feel the ache begin to ease.* This embodied "knowing" activates the parasympathetic system, and you will begin to relax and settle. Parasympathetic rest will allow your body to begin its own process of restorative self-repair. This is because all the major organ systems connected to the ANS, including the immune system, can relax and do their healing work.

Summary and Conclusions

This chapter has introduced the three states of embodied self-awareness and described how the nervous system supports four basic types of felt experience: interoceptive, proprioceptive, autonomic, and emotional. Although we can classify each of these experiences as separate and unique, and even though they arise from different pathways in the nervous system, they typically co-occur in different combinations depending on the situation.[29]

This is most likely because all feelings are not only brought into our ESA by passing through the insula, but the insula—often working with the ventromedial prefrontal cortex—serves the function of knitting together all the threads of experience into a single felt experience of embodiment.[30] Research studies conducted at the Universities of Lille and Lyon (France), and also at the Laureate Institute for Brain Research (Tulsa, Oklahoma, USA), show that people who test high on the autonomic awareness of their hearts beating are also highly attuned to other autonomic feelings such as gastric fullness and to different kinds of interoceptive sensations.[31] In this book, we'll be exploring the ways in which the many hundreds of such complex, integrated felt experiences can manifest in everyday life.

As we'll see in the next chapters, interoceptive, proprioceptive, emotional, or autonomic feelings are actually experienced differently in each state of ESA. The emotion of pleasure or enjoyment is one example that will be described in chapter 6 (see "Enjoyment/Pleasure," p. 191). Restorative pleasure comes with a sense of completeness, calm, and connection. Modulated pleasure is more like a moment of enjoyment that is felt with the successful completion of an ongoing activity. Modulated pleasure might also occur during laughter with other people as part of a shared accomplishment or amusement. Dysregulated pleasure accompanies the intake of some addictive substance or the perverse pleasure that some people may derive from harming themselves or others.

The language of the body in each state of ESA takes a while to feel and to understand. As you read what follows in the rest of this book, stay aware of your questions and your assumptions. See if you can keep yourself open and free to explore new ways of thinking about and feeling your embodied experience.

It may also help to keep an open focus of attention. Try slowing down and even stopping reading for a while, especially if you feel that you want to plow through the material or get done with the book or a particular chapter. The feeling of wanting to rush through may be a message from your body to give yourself time to let the information sink in, both into your conceptual ideas and into what you are feeling.

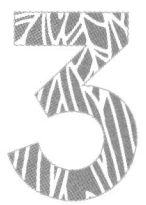

Three States of Embodied Self-Awareness

Felt Experience, Thinking, and Autonomic Nervous System Activation

In this chapter we'll take an in-depth look at each of the three states of ESA. For each state, there will be a description of the types of felt experience that can occur in that state, the types of thinking that characterize each state, and the activity of the autonomic nervous system for each state. There will also be examples that help ground each state in real-life experience.

Qualities of Restorative Embodied Self-Awareness

Restorative Felt Experience

Restorative ESA is the ability to fully embrace any felt experience—pleasure or pain, happiness or grief, hopefulness or despair—that may arise in the present moment without judgmental or censoring thoughts. Restorative feelings come with the sense of finding an inner truth about ourselves, what we "really" feel as opposed to what we think we feel.

This occurs when felt experience is sustained and entirely in the present moment. *Sustained* means that we give ourselves sufficient time for the experience to engender a lasting sense of relief, a deeper breath, a spreading feeling of warmth or relaxation (a primarily parasympathetic state with little or no sympathetic activation).[1]

Researchers in the Department of Public Health, Policy and Social Sciences at Swansea University (UK) reviewed the results of 237 research studies related to the links between the ANS and other forms of felt experience. They found a consistent pattern: people who showed greater acceptance of emotional felt experiences had higher levels of parasympathetic activation.[2]

Even if the felt experience is "negative"—like getting in touch with some pain, grief, or trauma—it becomes restorative once we feel, embrace, and accept it as a part of who we are: what we are honestly feeling in the moment and whatever may have happened to us in the past. Restorative felt experience comes with calmness, tranquility, clarity, and openness.[3] If you have any sense of control, planning, or effort, or if you do not feel any settling of your nervous system, then you are most likely in a state of modulated ESA.

- ◆ A felt experience is restorative *only* if it is accompanied or followed by *a felt parasympathetic state of rest.*

- ◆ Feelings that are restorative *only* come spontaneously and *without TPN (task-positive network) or DMN (default-mode network) conceptual thought* or focused attention or planning.

- Felt experience is restorative *only* if it has the quality of vividness, of filling up our awareness—in other words, *of our being fully present with the feeling.*[4]

- The *only* way to access restorative felt experience is by slowing down, letting go, surrendering to being fully in the moment, and allowing our attention to be broad and free-floating—in other words, *without "doing," effort, or deliberate control.*

Any kind of interoceptive, proprioceptive, emotional, or autonomic feeling—positive or negative, pleasurable or painful, exciting or boring—has the potential to be restorative so long as it meets these criteria. In later chapters, there will be many examples of what restorative experiences feel like and how they differ from modulated or dysregulated felt experiences. Right now, let's begin with some examples of felt experiences that can *only* occur during states of restorative ESA.

Awe, for example, is a sense of expansiveness, oneness, and completeness. It occurs typically in "spiritual" or "transcendent" experiences, such as when we come in contact with inspiring works of visual and performance art, in front of massive landscapes like mountains and oceans, or looking up at large human-made entities like skyscrapers, temples and houses of worship, pyramids, the Statue of Liberty, or the Eiffel Tower.[5] Religious experiences may also evoke a feeling of awe. Awe is often accompanied by parasympathetic body sensations such as chills, goose bumps, expansiveness in the breath and chest, and tears—not of sadness or pain but of wonder-joy.[6]

John M. de Castro of the Center for Mindfulness and Contemplative Studies (Huntsville, Texas, USA) and Michiel van Elk and his colleagues at the Brain and Cognition Center of the University of Amsterdam (the Netherlands) have shown that awe is fundamentally an experience of restorative ESA. First of all, awe experiences suppress activity in the dorsomedial prefrontal cortex and the default-mode network (DMN). This means that during awe, we are not occupied with self-related thoughts. Second, awe activates the ventromedial prefrontal cortex, which allows us to hold felt experience in the present moment for a sustained period of time.[7]

Awe is unlike many other kinds of positive emotional experiences such as feelings of pleasure, enthusiasm, and amusement. These emotions may sometimes happen in restorative ESA states, but they can also occur in both dysregulated and modulated ESA involving sympathetic arousal (e.g., jumping for joy; see chapter 6, "Enjoyment/Pleasure," p. 191). Awe, on the other hand, both suppresses sympathetic activity and increases parasympathetic activity in the body,[8] meaning that awe generates a state of relaxation, an absence of thinking, a lowering of arousal, and the feeling of being completely in the present moment.[9]

Aside from ushering us into states of relaxation, awe has been shown to have genuine restorative properties. Researchers from the University of California, Berkeley (USA), looked at the effects of a white water rafting wilderness adventure on people who had suffered trauma. Their sample consisted of seventy-four military veterans and fifty-two youth from underserved communities (38 percent female). The participants took either one-day or four-day rafting trips that were organized by the Sierra Club Outdoors organization during the 2015 and 2016 summer white water rafting seasons.

Researchers examined participants' daily diaries for each day of the trips, and they sent post-adventure questionnaires related to mental health and PTSD symptoms one week following the end of the trip. They found that not all of the participants experienced a sense of awe. Those participants whose diaries reported more awe experiences, however, showed significant improvements in mental health and reduction of self-reported trauma symptoms on the questionnaires filled out one week later.[10]

Like some of the participants in this study, not everyone feels awe while floating in the immense power of a fast-moving and turbulent river, surrounded by the forests and cliffs that contain and amplify the river's course and speed. Some people may be overwhelmed not with awe but with fear. When the untamed power of nature instills fear, it will activate fight, flight, or freeze responses. This can exacerbate the trauma symptoms such wilderness-therapy experiences might have been designed to address, keeping people in highly aroused states of dysregulated ESA.[11]

It is important, therefore, to distinguish the experience of awe from the particular settings where awe may be likely to occur. One can be walking along a beach bordered by impressive highlands and with waves crashing over rocks the size of houses, a cloudless sky above and soft sand below. In such a place, some people are more dispositionally predisposed to experience awe. Others, even if they are not feeling afraid, may take this same walk preoccupied with TPN or DMN thoughts related to things going on in their lives or else engaged in conversation with other people. The wave sounds and sea smells might come into awareness from time to time, but attention is focused on what is being said and thought. These people are trudging through the sand of modulated ESA.

Individuals who score high on tests of dispositional awe—compared to those who rarely have this experience or who are threatened by something that might potentially be awesome to someone else—score higher on measures of well-being. People high on dispositional awe also report that their lives have some kind of transcendent meaning beyond their everyday tasks and commitments; they care less about material possessions and more about a connection to spiritual experiences. These people show higher levels of concern and caring for other people individually and in the collective sense of sustaining humanity and the value of human life.[12]

It is curious that a tendency to be open to feeling awe creates not only well-being—which we would expect because of the restorative parasympathetic activation—but also the sense that human life has transcendent meaning. Awe is generated during experiences of being overtaken by something much larger than the self, by an amazement at the scope and power of nature and humanity, and by a sense of being in harmony and in oneness with the earth and its inhabitants.[13] Interview studies suggest that this creates a sense of a "small self," a self-transcendent feeling that we are part of something much larger than our own individuality.[14]

This idea of a small self does not mean that we think of ourselves as unimportant. In fact, during awe experiences, we are not thinking. Rather, it is like we melt away into a larger cosmos that is powerful and inspiring beyond measure. This also explains why people who more regularly experience awe are more likely to feel less attached to possessions and personal achievements. They see themselves as part of something bigger, something in which there is a sense of oneness and connection.[15]

Research at the Memory and Aging Center of the University of California, San Francisco (USA), looked at the effects of "awe walks" on fifty-three people in their sixties to eighties.[16] They were asked to take a fifteen-minute walk every day focusing on just being present with their surroundings and seeing everything "new," as if from a child's perspective. They were compared with a similar-age control group who was given no such instruction about how to walk. Both groups were interviewed and also asked to take selfies each day and send them to the lab.

The awe walkers developed an ability to really notice their surroundings and connect with the colors, sounds, and smells. The control-group walkers, on the other hand, reporting using their walking time in DMN thoughts and worries about all they had to do. The study lasted eight weeks, and over the course of that time, surprising the researchers, selfies of the awe walkers showed a gradual reduction in the size of the person in the picture compared to their surroundings. They literally became smaller selves! No such effect happened in the control group.

Additionally, questionnaires revealed that the awe walkers showed increases in well-being, feelings of happiness, and social connection compared with the control group. Other similar research has shown that feelings of oneness with nature and other people are also associated with measures of well-being and life satisfaction.[17]

Another felt experience that can occur only in restorative states is a sense of safety and contentment. Scientists at the Mental Health Research Unit of Kingsway Hospital (Derby, UK) showed that the higher people score on measures of felt safety, the lower their scores on some of the characteristics of dysregulated ESA such as depression, anxiety, stress, and self-critical DMN ruminations.[18] A higher felt sense of safety and contentment is associated with higher activation of the parasympathetic nervous system[19] and is also connected with the ability to fully access embodied felt experience without intervening thought.[20]

As we shall see in this book, many other kinds of experiences can be restorative so long as they meet the criteria listed at the beginning of this section. We shall also see that thinking, especially in modulated ESA states, can convince us that we are having a restorative experience when, in fact, the important facets of restoration are not actually occurring because thinking puts us into a sympathetic state.

And the paradox of restorative felt experience is that, as explained in the following section, it does not involve any kind of meaning-making thought: when we are actually in a restorative ESA state, we don't know we are in it, if by "knowing" we mean that we can in some way explain or understand it. And conversely, if we think we know we are in a restorative state, then we are most likely in a modulated state using our TPN thinking.

In that sense, restorative experience is neither predictable nor modulated. We can't control it. We surrender to it. Like riding a wave, we allow the experience to take us in its own way and in its own time.[21] Restorative felt experience is itself awesome because we lose ourselves in it (we become a small self) and at the same time we find ourselves: what we really feel, what is true for us, our true self.[22]

Restorative Thought

There is thought during states of restorative ESA, but that thought is not rational, logical, or directed, nor is it organized into linguistic sentences. Restorative thought is without any narrative content and is not produced by either the TPN or the DMN. You are probably wondering what kind of thought this might be, or if it even is possible.

Restorative thought may consist of words, sounds, images, and vivid memories that are not accompanied by any form of explanation. Instead, these types of thought arise spontaneously in relation to the particular felt experience in the present moment.[23] The key to thoughts being restorative is that they serve to amplify or deepen the felt experience rather than take us away from that experience.

Nonconceptual, nonlogical thoughts can take many forms. There might, for example, be a thought of a single word or a series of words that are "evocative,"[24] meaning that they amplify or resonate with a felt experience. Evocative words "touch" us, create in us an emotional response that might bring tears or anger. Evocative words happen when we think of something or when someone says something to us that is heartfelt or hurtful, that reaches a deep place inside of us of a genuine felt experience.

Evocative words can come in the form of a poem, play, novel, song, or speech that can connect to or open up a restorative felt experience inside ourselves. While it is true that these examples all contain linguistic sentences, it is not the logic of the words that moves us but rather the emotional impact the words have on us. Song, poetry, theater, film, literature, and storytelling all use words for the purpose of communicating the full range of human emotions, for getting us in touch with our feelings. If words "reach us," they are felt as true, deep, powerful, and fundamentally restorative.

Evocative language, language that reaches and moves those who read or listen, can only arise from a person who speaks, writes, or sings directly from an unguarded and vulnerable openness to their own feelings. Such words have the power to change us, to give us inner vision, to deepen our inner clarity of our current woes and possibilities, to heighten our embodied awareness as a participant in a fully alive and deeply gratifying human condition.

When we are thinking in the form of on-task or off-task narratives, the linguistic areas of the brain mentioned in chapter 1 (areas for hearing, vision, and speech comprehension and production, Figure 1.4, p. 17) are connected directly to the brain's TPN and DMN (Figures 1.3, p. 15, and 1.5, p. 21). When words are evocative and restorative, on the other hand, these same linguistic areas become disconnected from the TPN and DMN and instead are directly connected to the networks for felt experience via the insula and the ventromedial prefrontal cortex. Words that describe movements, for example, show increased activation in the insula and ventromedial prefrontal cortex as well as in the sensorimotor cortex, accompanied by a suppression of activation in the TPN and DMN.[25]

Evocative words and sounds *arise spontaneously* in awareness and do not come from a directed or focused thought process. Having a broad and free-floating form of attention, as opposed to focused attention, also disconnects the DMN and reroutes consciousness into present-moment felt experience.[26] This kind of open attention—and its associated thought and language—has been described in certain forms of meditation, in psychoanalytic free association, in composing music and poetry, and in some spiritual traditions.[27] A broad form of attention has also been associated with higher levels of felt happiness and contentment.[28]

In one research study done at the Brain and Creativity Institute (University of Southern California, Los Angeles, USA), people were asked to listen to several different kinds of narratives related to compassion, virtue, skill, and personal experiences. After listening, they were asked to describe for each of the narratives, "How does this person's story make you feel?" Participants differed in their use of words, some choosing to respond to this question using "cognitive" words and others choosing to respond using "emotion" words.

Examples of cognitive words are *think, know, assume, should,* and *acknowledge*—that is, words reflecting types of thought typically generated in the TPN and DMN. Emotion words included *happy, inspiring, crying, abandon,* and *cruel.* People who used the emotion language showed higher activation in the emotional felt-experience areas of the brain: in the insula, anterior cingulate cortex, and sensorimotor areas (see Figure 2.5, p. 68).[29]

Words are not the only kind of restorative thought that can occur. Restorative thoughts can be composed of sounds—like "hearing" inside ourselves bells ringing, waves lapping, a loved one's voice, or certain types of music.[30] Nonverbal sounds (grunting from effort, expressions of elation or frustration) made during athletics or dance movements can also have evocative effects on the felt experiences of both the performer and the observer.[31]

Visual mental images—a loved one's face, a scene of natural beauty, aesthetic experiences of art or architecture, a familiar and comforting room or other location—may have evocative-restorative effects including increased parasympathetic activation, lower levels of cortisol, suppression of amygdala activity, and enhanced activity in the ventromedial prefrontal cortex, and thus suppression of the DMN and TPN.[32]

Restorative thought can also come in the form of vivid memories that are "alive," composed not of narrative stories but of visual images or sensory experiences. These remembrances could be happy ones, such as touching or being touched, or of moving one's body in a restorative way, such as dancing or walking, or of doing something athletic or artistic, or of an intimate encounter with another person. They could also be troubling or traumatic memories that evoke particular emotions and sensations in our felt experience. These recollections are called *participatory memories,* meaning that we have the felt sense of reliving an experience in the present moment, more like a dream than an autobiographical story-narrative.[33]

Participatory memories, and imagined future scenarios that are similarly alive or vivid, occur when the ventromedial prefrontal cortex is activated and the dorsomedial prefrontal cortex, TPN, and DMN are suppressed.[34] When we experience vivid, emotional, participatory memories, the ventromedial prefrontal cortex becomes linked to the amygdala and to the hippocampus (a semicircular structure that goes around the inside of the mid-brain, roughly directly behind and on both sides of the nose), the parts of the brain that create and give access to emotionally salient past experiences.[35]

In the formation of autobiographical narrative memories, the hippocampus is more closely linked to the TPN, DMN, and language centers of the brain, and not to the more present-moment felt experiences related to the ventromedial prefrontal cortex. There is some sympathetic effort involved in constructing the story-narrative, whether we are sharing the memory verbally with others or just thinking about the memory in logically connected sentences that make up the story about the remembered experience. The same is true if the imagined future takes a linguistic-narrative form. When we "look forward" to something, to take one example, not only is there mental effort but typically also muscle tension in the upper body and around the head and eyes. It is as if we are straining to see something that we want to happen or wanting to make it happen sooner.

Restorative thought has sometimes been connected to the concept of the "true self." One research study done at the Rotman School of Management, University of Toronto (Canada), for example, found that people differ on how they make choices, such as whether to buy one or another DVD player, or one of several different types of insulated drinking mugs, which restaurant they might go to, or which of four apartments they might rent. Some people used their felt experience while others use their TPN and DMN thinking to evaluate those choices. Those who used their felt experience considered themselves to be closer to their "true self." According to the authors of this study, the idea of the true self is something that is believed

> *to be situated at an inwardly deep and core, fundamental level,*
> *and is where resides the essence of the individual ... It is contrasted*
> *with how the actual self might outwardly, waveringly think or act*

depending on different situations … a more strongly felt connection with this true self as the force guiding choices makes life seem more meaningful … and enables better and more satisfying decisions.[36]

In contrast to the true self, when our sense of ourselves comes from our TPN and DMN thoughts, it can mislead us into thinking we want or need a particular thing, what the psychiatrist Donald Winnicott calls the "false self." According to Winnicott, there is a

tie-up between the intellectual approach and the False Self … and in this case there develops a dissociation between intellectual activity and psycho-somatic existence … The True Self comes from the aliveness of the body tissues and the working of the body-functions, including the heart's action and breathing.[37]

In this research study, people whose product choices were based on feelings rather than on thinking felt themselves closer to their true self. Their decisions were imbued with a greater sense of certainty, and they were more willing to stand up for those decisions and advocate on behalf of those choices.

Another research study done at the School of Business Administration, University of Wisconsin–Milwaukee (USA), looked at how people made career choices. People who used "rational"—that is, TPN—strategies to choose among different job opportunities had a reasonable level of success in finding a job that matched their abilities and expectations. An example of a rational strategy was, "I made sure the decision was based on much careful thought and deliberation."

If, however, people used an "intuitive" strategy instead of a rational approach, the match between themselves and their job was even higher. An example of this approach is, "I based my decision on whether it felt emotionally satisfying to me." Again, our felt experiences about choices, rather than thinking, bring us closer to the gut feelings of the true self.[38]

In summary, restorative thought does not originate from the TPN or DMN. It is not logical. It is not a narrative or story. It does not take us away from felt experience but rather brings us right back to our embodied feelings. Restorative thought "rings" or resonates inside of us, inside the whole body, and brings us closer to our true self.

Restorative Autonomic Nervous System

Restoration *always* coincides with activation of the ventral vagal parasympathetic and the dorsal vagal parasympathetic "immobilization without fear" nervous systems, which yields a natural and easy breath, sighs, feeling slowed down, relaxation of muscular tension/armoring, relief, feelings of restoration, spreading warmth/energy, feeling soothed, safe, seen, held, settled, vulnerable, open, content, peaceful, fully present, and fully alive.[39] As one example, feelings of oneness and awe, described earlier in this section on qualities of restorative ESA, correlate with measures of higher levels of parasympathetic activation.[40] Parasympathetic activation also creates a state of *homeostasis*, the ability of the body's functional systems (the immune, hormonal, respiratory, urinary, reproductive, sexual, digestive, and cardiovascular systems) to be sufficiently resilient to recover and provide whole-body restoration of health.[41]

As with research on awe, there are individual differences. Certain people seek out and value experiences that evoke a feeling of parasympathetic calmness; others seek experiences that arouse sympathetic feelings of excitement, such as amusement park rides, high-intensity exercise like rock climbing or Zumba, or competitive sports.[42] As described in the following two sections, engagement in high-arousal sympathetic activity may occur during states of modulated or dysregulated ESA, depending upon one's sense of control vs. compulsion.

Qualities of Modulated Embodied Self-Awareness

Modulated Felt Experience

Felt experiences in states of modulated ESA have all the same components of those in restorative ESA: interoceptive, proprioceptive, autonomic, and emotional feelings. The difference is that these experiences are transient rather than sustained. Modulated felt experience is typically a brief moment of feeling that is part of keeping busy, engaged, or creative.

Brief felt experiences may include moments of grounding, reconnecting, or coming back to oneself but only as a short break from ongoing activity and not as a sustained awareness. We can stop, get up from where we were sitting, stretch, rub our shoulders, play with the dog, refill our cup or glass, go to the bathroom, take a few deep breaths, or whatever else we like to do that helps us reconnect with our body. These activities, however, happen against the background of a need to keep working on a task with only a relatively brief pause.

Using modulated thought (see next section), we are exerting some kind of deliberate and focused control over what we are doing, including making the conscious choice to slow down a bit. We are keeping track of the time, monitoring how long we can afford to take a break, making decisions about how to get tasks accomplished while still taking care of ourselves and our bodily needs.

In this modulated state, however, most of the time we are not aware of the felt experiences arising in our body. Our awareness is almost entirely focused on our sensorimotor actions related to what we are doing and/or on our TPN or DMN thinking. Most of the time, most of us are in this state, and it usually feels alive, productive, helpful, creative; but it can also feel intense and too much and can sometimes transform into dysregulated ESA.

In modulated felt experience, we move in and out of brief feelings, staying on the "edge" of potentially deeper experiences of restorative ESA (which is why we can't reach a felt experience such as awe in a state of modulated ESA). At the same time, our self-modulation is also keeping us from getting lost into dysregulated states. We somehow get that if we push ourselves too hard, work without breaks, and don't take care of our basic needs for nourishment and rest, that we will get stressed out, irritable, overtired, or burned out.

Modulated Thought

Modulated ESA is a state in which thought, rather than feeling, is predominant. In TPN mode, our thoughts are purposeful or intentional. They are conceptual, deliberate, categorical, and adaptive to the situation. This generative task-focused thought can include creative thinking and problem solving, decision making, explaining, understanding, planning, or thoughts about self and others that are not obsessive but move toward a specific goal such as telling a story or collaborating with other people on reaching a particular shared goal.

We might be planning a project at work. We might be organizing our children to get up, dressed, fed, and off to school. We might be solving mathematical problems, or writing computer programs, or creating a product in manufacturing or agriculture or food service. We might be figuring out how to get something done on one of our devices. We might we be organizing a social gathering. We might be working with a customer, supervisor, or employee. We might be planning a vacation.

If we are members of a vulnerable or minority group, we are likely to be very focused on modulating our relationship to the environment around us. We might need to think about where we walk or run, where we take our children, how we dress, talk, or present ourselves so as to not attract attention to our gender status, our skin color, our religion, or our ethnicity. Or we might be thinking about how to emphasize and take pride in our particular identity. Whatever we choose about how to be in the world, we are forced into staying in a modulated state with little room for restoration. Do we wear garments that identify us as members of a religious or ethnic group? Do we show cleavage or wear tight-fitting clothing in a professional meeting? Are we Black and proud or Black and terrified? Are we white and ignorant of our privilege, or are we white and thinking about how we create inequalities and bias?

We might be a person with some kind of sensorimotor disability. We might have mental health issues. We might be under treatment for a chronic condition like cancer or awaiting an organ transplant. We might be a refugee seeking asylum. Having to deal with these issues every day, to solve basic problems of mobility and self-presentation, takes sympathetic arousal and near-constant thought.

From the perspective of ESA, the content and context of the sympathetic arousal do not matter. Our dorsomedial prefrontal cortex, DMN, and TPN are doing most of the work while the ventromedial prefrontal cortex, insula, and other circuits for felt experience are relatively suppressed. Even during our modulated breaks and pauses, it is highly likely that our DMN—and not our felt experience—becomes more active as the TPN focus fades into the background. Like the TPN, the DMN suppresses our ability to connect with felt experience.

During modulated ESA, when we are doing any of the re-grounding activities mentioned in the previous section, we are only minimally paying attention to felt experience. Our DMN is reviewing, revisiting, churning through what has occurred in the recent past, and this keeps us from dropping into a deeper parasympathetic and, therefore, restorative felt experience.

Here's the voice of the DMN: "How did I do with that constant male and female gaze at my (cis or trans) female body? Did I make a good or bad impression? Did I keep myself and my family safe when we were out of the house? Was I a good enough parent today? Did I make all those calls or send all those emails to the people I wanted to connect with? Did I get enough exercise or drink enough water or have too much alcohol or food?" It's endless, this running inner commentary of questions.

Of course, while restorative ESA is essential for health and well-being, modulated on- and off-task thinking is essential for success in self-control, self-regulation, our everyday lives, jobs, and duties. While broad and unfocused attention is fundamental to the nondirected and open state of relaxation in restorative ESA, the focused attention that goes along with thinking through everyday life issues is crucial to being productive, making decisions, staying connected to people in satisfying and supportive ways, and staying safe in a potentially dangerous world.

But, as we learned in the previous section, relying entirely on thinking to make important decisions has some risk because we may be completely ignoring our gut feelings. In the "best" kind of modulated state, we can tap momentarily into those gut feelings—the true self—as a way to put the logical, thinking, decision-making process into a more embodied perspective. There is another risk, however, which is that we can approach our emotions via a thought process that avoids or skirts the actual or "true" emotion.

EMOTIONAL INTELLIGENCE

One example of the potential subversion of the true self is the cultivation of the skill of emotional intelligence. Emotional intelligence is about our ability to use our TPN and DMN to perceive, understand, and express in words our current emotional state, as well as recognizing and being able to name the emotional states of other people. Emotional intelligence relies on thinking strategies to regulate intense emotional experiences. When stressed or anxious, afraid or sad, we can use thinking to remind ourselves that these are just feelings, that we can let them happen, and that they will pass in time.

Success in applying emotional intelligence to one's life is measured by self-report scales that have items in the TPN realm. These items include "I have a good sense of why I have certain feelings most of the time," "I always know whether or not I am happy," "I understand the emotions of people around me," and "I can control my temper and handle difficulties."

It's important to acknowledge that emotional intelligence can be a wonderful skill to attain, particularly if we have been relatively ignorant of our emotional states. People who score high on emotional intelligence measures are also healthier and make choices to stay healthy, such as eating wellness-promoting foods, taking appropriate medications, exercising, brushing and flossing, and noticing changes in health status.[43]

People who use emotional intelligence to notice and accept that they are in a state of stress are more resilient: able to recover and restabilize to help prevent slipping into dysregulated states of ruminative worry. When using one's emotional intelligence while in a state of modulated ESA, what seems to help the most for diminishing dysregulated/ruminative worry is thinking about problem solving—using our TPN and DMN to figure out a way to reduce the need for worry while anticipating and learning to avoid future worrisome episodes.[44]

For example, research conducted by the US Department of Veterans Affairs on 2,157 returned combat veterans who were exposed to traumatic wartime events shows that the veterans differ on whether they later develop symptoms of post-traumatic stress disorder. The more resilient veterans who are physically healthier, who do not engage in substance abuse, and who have reasonably good emotional intelligence and self-modulating skills are more outgoing and altruistic. They feel their lives have a purpose, and they are less likely to develop PTSD.[45]

Clearly, modulated TPN and DMN thinking that is (like emotional intelligence) devoted to the understanding of body states and emotions confers a protective advantage against both physical and mental disorders. People who are higher on scores of emotional intelligence are less likely to engage in dysregulated risk taking that threatens health and physical safety, such as unprotected sex, drunk driving, eating disorders, and so on.[46]

So, like all forms of modulated ESA, emotional intelligence is good for us and keeps us from getting into unhealthy and dysregulated states. But there is an inherent paradox: conceptual thought in modulated ESA—and the kinds of thoughts related to emotional intelligence—has the limitation that we are thinking about emotional feelings rather than directly accessing the felt experience.

In fact, some research done at the Universities of Worcester and Manchester (UK) has shown that emotional intelligence, while helpful in forming an immediate coping response to stress, has a limited ability to change the physiological components of the stress response. Although emotional intelligence can use thought processes to keep us sitting in a dental chair during uncomfortable procedures or pushing through challenges at work or in a sports activity, it does little to control a racing heart rate, rapid breathing, or fearful or anxious feelings.[47] The most effective way to shift our physiology from a state of high arousal into a state of relaxation is to drop into the possibly uncomfortable felt experience of that physiology to find restorative, parasympathetic states.

Thinking about a feeling may include thoughts such as "I must feel happy because I'm smiling," "I'm really sorry for what I did—I was not considerate," or "You think I look sad? I guess so, because I missed that opportunity." Or we might be seeking explanations about a momentary, modulated felt experience, like "Why am I feeling happy (sad, angry) right now? I'm sure there is an explanation. Maybe because of what my boss said to me?"

When we are thinking in these ways about felt experience, we can fool ourselves that we are actually feeling something. In modulated ESA, there is a nearly constant stream of conceptual thought that is so pervasive, so part of everyday life, that we might not even notice it. The brief moments of felt experience that can occur in modulated ESA may "stand out" against the background of thinking and *make us think* we are more present with our feelings than we actually are.

We can also use thinking to convince ourselves or another person that feeling is not needed, or that we are feeling something when we are not, or that we feel OK and can keep going (even though, if we took the time to find and feel our true self, we might encounter exhaustion or frustration or resentment). Modulated ESA, in other words, is a reasonably well-regulated state of thinking, keeping us functional, and it lives somewhere in between restorative and dysregulated ESA.

Modulated ESA is also the state we are living in most of the time. Rational, logical, task-oriented thinking is such a powerful way to meet the challenges of the world, a trait only found in humans. From an evolutionary perspective over millennia, as the outer layers of the brain grew bigger and held more capacity for thought, language, and creative problem solving, the human body developed a priority system for allocating metabolic energy to the thinking parts of the brain and away from the felt experiences and energy needs of the rest of the body.[48]

That's all great, uniquely human, and, in most cases, highly adaptive. But this thinking and rerouting of our metabolism come at a cost. Any kind of repression of felt experience, whether modulated or dysregulated, will lower blood glucose, compromise the immune system, and increase the risk of allergies, cancers, and other immune-depletion disorders.[49]

In other words, if we are challenged by everyday or urgent tasks and responsibilities, *we are preprogrammed to route glucose, lactate, and fatty-acid energy sources to the thought centers of the brain and away from sustaining the basic functions of the living body.* Our body may feel exhausted, our muscles may ache, our stomach may hurt, our eyes and ears may be strained, our immune system may be compromised to the point of illness—all of that and still we will continue to think!

Modulated Autonomic Nervous System

Modulated ESA activates primarily sympathetic pathways to maintain arousal and engagement. Thinking takes energy and the activation of internal organ systems in much the same way as does physical exercise. Hyperactive sympathetic activation, where we can't slow down, is a marker of dysregulated ESA. In modulated ESA, in contrast, we have the ability to feel when we are getting tired or moody or frustrated: we have the possibility to notice and take self-care measures because we can detect, even briefly, the metabolic and hormonal drain of sympathetic activation.

If we are modulated, it means we can slow down at least enough to activate brief moments of parasympathetic relaxation. This opens our eyes and our blood vessels, activates our digestive system to function normally, slows the production of cortisol, allows us to absorb nutrients and open the urinary and rectal sphincter muscles so that we can eliminate waste buildup, and gives at least a small opening for felt experience.

Assuming we are reasonably healthy, there is nothing wrong with being sympathetically activated for most of the day. In fact, this is the state of the ANS we are accustomed to living in. We need to make a living. We need to bring up our children. We need to protect ourselves and family from dangers. We need stimulation, exercise, and creative activities. The felt experience of autonomic activation is primarily aroused, excited, "up," rapid pulse and respiration, intensity, and being busy.

Resilience is the ability to use modulated activities to recover from states of dysregulated ESA. Generally, we can modulate the ANS with exercise, focused mindfulness meditation, eating well, indulging in outings with friends, going to cultural events, or having a fun weekend or a needed vacation. These activities all help diminish dysregulated feelings of stress, overwhelm, and burnout.[50]

GOING WITH THE FLOW

One highly rewarding aspect of modulated ESA is being in a state of "flow." In flow, we feel totally engaged, in the moment, at the unique intersection of our best abilities as we engage with other people, with our work, and with our artistic, musical, athletic, culinary, or other activities. These are peak experiences that occur when what we are called upon to do brings us to the highest level of our skill and performance. We are totally immersed in the felt experience of our body performing the perfect swimming or tennis stroke, sewing a garment, preparing a satisfying meal, playing a musical instrument, singing, dancing, or being with another person.

Flow is an almost purely sympathetically aroused state. Even though we may be completely in touch with our felt experience during the flow state, we are definitely not relaxed. We are at the outer limits of our abilities, moving and sensing, which requires all of our available metabolic, autonomic, and hormonal resources.

Flow is an example of what has been called **eustress**, a sympathetic state of arousal that activates and actually enhances our psychophysiological resources. If we are able to feel the arousal associated with challenging activities—at home, at work, or in leisure time—we are more likely to accept and modulate these experiences.

Eustress—the ability to remain open and engaged with new and challenging experiences—improves cardiovascular and hormonal responses, making us more resilient to everyday stressors.[51] Exercise is another example of eustress because it builds cardiovascular fitness and muscle strength, allowing us to run or walk longer distances or become better at sports. Eustress is a way of seeing stress as part of a desired outcome or activity, a sympathetic state that can be beneficial.

In these states of modulated flow or eustress, we are accessing the sense of feeling alive and connected to ourselves. Imagine performing music, theater, or athletics in front of a large audience where you are putting your total self, everything that you have, on the line.

In a study done in the Department of Music and Department of Sports at the University of Ljubljana (Slovenia), of 452 elite musicians and top athletes, this experience of the body engaging in these advanced skills at the "perfect" level of challenge was shown to enhance overall feelings of satisfaction with life. Researchers from the Cambridge Biomedical Research Centre (University of Cambridge, UK) found that among London stock market floor traders working daily in high-financial-risk situations, the most successful traders were the most attuned to their felt experience and most satisfied with their abilities.[52]

We may also feel the compulsion to create, compete, win, or be brilliant in front of other people. In these kinds of situations, there is often an element of fear, tension, danger, or pressure connected with living at the edge of our ability. There is a limit to how much of this our body can process. Many elite performers become dysregulated by the intensity and frequency of engaging in such experiences, often turning to drugs, sexual promiscuity, or alcohol as an attempt to manage the pressure.

Most likely your sewing project or meal preparation is not as risky as the performances of professional athletes, musicians, or stock traders. But you still have an "audience" of family and friends who eat the meal or see the garment you have constructed. So, as you work on your project, your imaginary audience is adding an element of sympathetically aroused pressure.

The risks you take may be small, like how much pepper or sweetness or salt is going to make your food stand out and elicit compliments. In the middle of the peak experience, it may seem like the activity will last forever. It doesn't, of course, because we run out of gas; we need to slow down and rest. At these times, when this peak moment has subsided, we have the possibility to arrive at a more complete state of rest in restorative ESA, like sinking into an altered state of consciousness when lying together with a partner after making love or finding peace and rest in the Corpse pose after an intense yoga workout.

For genuine restoration to happen, we have to give in and surrender to the feeling of letting go of all the energy and tension. Or maybe we remain in a state of modulated ESA. Our sympathetic nervous system continues to burn even after the activity, and instead of finding a complete state of rest, we have brief moments of parasympathetic letdown, and then we transition into DMN thoughts about all the things we did right or wrong, or that we still have to do or say.

Our lovemaking or meal sharing or yoga workout can be a peak experience followed by a few moments of calm, but we continue to remain mentally and physiologically aroused and are quick to get up and move on to the next task. There will be more about noticing and optimizing how we shift between states of ESA in the next chapters.

Too little stimulation or challenge can feel tedious or boring. Too much can feel edgy, vigilant, tense, excessive, or driven to the point of confusion, distraction, fatigue, withdrawal. Even with these more "negative" feelings, being modulated means that we are able to activate brief parasympathetic re-grounding and refreshing. We can take a break. We can think about how to find the sweet spot or the groove of flow where we can discover the best of ourselves in action.

Qualities of Dysregulated Embodied Self-Awareness

Dysregulation means that we cannot stop, we are stuck, we cannot help ourselves, we cannot change our felt experience or its intensity, we cannot rid ourselves of negative thoughts, and we cannot modulate our level of ANS arousal. There is no space to breathe, no rest, no relief. The painful and disturbing feelings and thoughts of dysregulated ESA are what usually lead people either to get help or into self-destructive measures that seem to ease the suffering, such as addiction, self-harm, overt hostility, or even suicide.[53]

Dysregulated Felt Experience

Dysregulated felt experience can take two forms. One form is a nearly constant and uncontrollable self-focus on feelings of acute and chronic states of physical and emotional discomfort, pain, fatigue, depression, and/or anxiety.

Depressive feelings include hopelessness, desperation, and despair, as well as feelings of uncomfortable self-consciousness such as chronic shame, self-doubt, and self-blame. Anxious feelings consist of being afraid and hypervigilant, having chronic muscle tension, and showing other physical symptoms like chest pains, shortness of breath, headaches, and stomachaches.

In research done at the Emory University School of Medicine (Atlanta, Georgia, USA), up to 25 percent of patients admitted to an emergency room for apparent heart attack were suffering instead from panic attacks, typically due to a recent episode of stress or trauma that affected stress-related brain areas (the amygdala and hypothalamus) and altered ANS activity related to the heart.[54] Many of the patients in this group had already suffered from some form of heart disease, which is likely to have contributed to their disturbing somatic symptoms of panic—symptoms that do, in fact, feel very much like a heart attack.[55]

And, conversely, having an anxiety disorder is stressful for the cardiovascular system and is linked to a hypersensitivity (a dysregulated felt experience) of any kind of chest pain or shortness of breath that might lead people to believe that they are having a heart, rather than a panic, attack.[56] This is another example of how "mind" and "body" are inseparable and how felt experiences "in the head," such as panic and worry, are mirrored and co-regulated with felt experiences in the rest of the body.

Another form of dysregulated felt experience consists of perverse and often destructive or harmful ways to make ourselves feel better. Some people resort to the "high" of risk taking, which makes them feel invulnerable. This might be driving too fast or recklessly, jumping off a cliff into a body of water, being sexually promiscuous, or getting into physical fights.

You might think that finding this high is a form of modulated flow experience. This is actually the opposite of what happens. Research at the University of Texas at Austin (USA) and the University of California, Los Angeles (USA), shows that these risks occur in high states of sympathetic activation in which ventromedial prefrontal cortex activity is suppressed.[57] Recall from Figure 2.1 (p. 52) that the ventromedial prefrontal cortex is the part of the brain that allows us to sustain, feel, and modulate felt experience. In the types of risk-taking situations described here, people are actually avoiding their painful felt experiences by substituting the high of being out of control to the point of endangering others and themselves, scaring people around them, and just acting "crazy."

Addictions are also ways to disconnect from uncomfortable feelings by enabling the feeling of being high. Because of the predictable emotional swings from discomfort to euphoria, addictions are forms of dysregulated felt experience that give the illusion of self-modulating.[58]

People who use, assault, or are overtly hostile to others who are younger, weaker, or more vulnerable are asserting a sense of power or control as a way to avoid their own feelings of loss, pain, loneliness, grief, or shame. To that person, these actions may seem like a kind of modulation of their intense painful experiences. But because the actions bring harm to self and others, they create the illusion of modulation when, in fact, the person is not able to stop and evaluate their actions. This is the definition of being dysregulated.

All these forms of avoidance of felt experience during chronically dysregulated states of ESA are dangerous for our self-integrity and for our physical and mental health and well-being. Chronic dysregulated ESA, such as with long-term and untreated anxiety or depression, actually carries a high risk of serious physical illness such as cardiovascular disease, diabetes, cancer, or digestive and respiratory ailments. The percentage of people with chronic dysregulated ESA who fall into these serious illness states is actually higher than the percentage of people who get life-threatening diseases from the usual culprits of obesity and smoking![59]

The kinds of dysregulated felt experiences described here have been linked to impairments in interoceptive, proprioceptive, autonomic, and emotional processing.[60] This kind of impairment of felt experience shows up across a broad range of illnesses including anxiety, depression, obsessive-compulsive disorder, chronic fatigue syndrome, fibromyalgia, and irritable bowel syndrome.[61]

These dysregulated impairments in felt experience related to illness conditions appear to be mediated by alterations of neurotransmitters and connections both within the insula and between the insula and other brain areas for felt experience.[62] Research done across several universities in Chile and the UK, and with individuals having different forms of physical and mental illness, clearly shows that the resulting dysregulated interoceptive experiences of the body have the quality of being unbearably intrusive.[63] Research done at Leiden University and the Free University of Amsterdam (the Netherlands) shows that children who had a higher number of complaints about somatic symptoms (headache, stomachache, dizziness, fatigue, nausea, shakiness) were more likely to report feeling negative emotions such as fear, sadness, and anger.[64]

DYSREGULATED LOSS IN AGING (AND PATHWAYS TOWARD RESTORATION)

For some individuals, the process of aging can create unwanted forms of dysregulated ESA. The peripheral receptors and unmyelinated conduction pathways to the brain regions that create felt experience become even more "leaky" as we age. It is a common observation that many older adults have difficulty with motor tasks and sometimes need supportive aids like walkers, canes, and wheelchairs. Urinary and bowel control can become compromised.

Although some of this is due to diminished muscle strength and tone, these deficits are caused primarily by impaired interoception and proprioception. The feelings from the periphery of the body become more attenuated as we age. People are less able to feel bladder fullness or to feel and control urinary muscles, which leads to incontinence. Locomotion challenges arise in a diminished ability to feel proprioceptive balance or parts of the lower legs and feet.

Interventions that give older adults practice moving and feeling can be helpful in restoring lost felt experience. There are many exercise classes such as water aerobics that promote mobility and strength for older adults. Classes that emphasize slow movement with awareness—such as Rosen Method Movement, Feldenkrais Awareness through Movement, dance/movement therapy, gentle (yin) yoga, or tai chi—provide enhanced proprioception of movement coordination, posture, and balance and reduce the risk of falling.[65] Yoga classes can also help with posture and body awareness. Similarly, exercises for feeling and practicing moving urinary and rectal muscles can help alleviate incontinence symptoms.

Some older adults may become more highly attuned to dysregulated feelings of pain and discomfort, which then diminishes their ability to sense their emotional and autonomic feelings. The reduced emotional awareness means that they rely more on external cues, especially other people's responses, to determine what or how they should feel in a particular situation. Impaired emotional felt awareness is part of what makes the elderly particularly susceptible to scams and other exploitations by strangers, friends, and family members.[66] These deficits in felt experience are even more pronounced in people with stroke, dementia, and Alzheimer's disease.[67]

It is not news that the elderly have more difficulty with proprioception, interoception, and movement (not to mention cognitive declines). What is important from the perspective of this book is that these types of impairments can be partly explained by factors related to dysfunction in the felt-experience neural networks of ESA. The good news is that education, embodied practices, and regular cognitive and physical exercises can help alleviate many of these conditions.

Dysregulated Thought

As in modulated ESA, dysregulated ESA is filled up with thinking. The thought patterns in each of these two states of ESA, however, are radically different. Modulated thought is productive and creative. It accomplishes tasks and goals, brings us a clearer sense of ourselves and other people, and helps us self-regulate when we sense that we are becoming more dysregulated. Modulated ESA thought is formed in the TPN (on-task thinking) and the DMN (off-task thinking).

In states of dysregulated ESA, TPN types of goal-directed and problem-solving thoughts are not available to us. At its core, being dysregulated means that we cannot solve our own problems and we see no way out; we are caught or trapped in negativity, pain, and/or decidedly unproductive and nonlogical decisions that lead us into risk and danger.

The salient theme of all DMN thought is an almost exclusive focus on the self and about how the self relates to other people and things in the world. In modulated ESA states, the posterior cingulate cortex works together with the regulatory dorsomedial prefrontal cortex to evoke thought that allows us to fill in the blanks and pick up the pieces of problems and concerns that—in our busy, mostly TPN daily thoughts—we missed or forgot (see Figures 1.3, p. 15, and 1.4, p. 17). The modulated DMN gives us a way to review the day or week, to remember and reconstruct, to make a mental list of things still left to be accomplished.

Dysregulated thinking arises not in the TPN but rather in a dysregulated DMN. Conditions that compromise body function, such as illness, stress, and trauma, set up the physiological conditions for dysregulation by triggering the amygdala to alert other brain areas to a sense of danger or threat. In the DMN, stress reduces the connectivity between the posterior cingulate cortex and modulating role of the dorsomedial prefrontal cortex (see Figure 1.5, p. 21).

When the dorsomedial prefrontal cortex goes off-line, so to speak, the result is that the self-focusing thinking in the DMN neural network is composed of the kinds of stuck, ruminative, and unproductive thoughts mentioned previously.[68] The self-enlightening functions of the modulated DMN become displaced by self-doubt, self-criticism, endless questions, worrying, defending, denying, depressive and self-negative thoughts, suicidal thoughts, hostile, blaming (self and other) and judgmental thought patterns (good/bad), mental confusion, and disorientation. Dysregulated DMN thoughts tend to co-occur with dysregulated felt experiences and dysregulated behavior.[69] We are stuck in them as they repeat in seemingly endless, ruminative loops.

An example of this comes from a study—done by researchers in the Department of Psychology, Yonsei University (Seoul, South Korea)—of 195 adult residents of Gyeongju and Pohang, coastal cities in South Korea where major earthquakes had occurred. The participants completed questionnaires assessing emotional clarity, emotion regulation, and post-traumatic stress symptoms a year and ten months after the Gyeongju earthquake and seven months after the Pohang earthquake. The earthquake survivors from both cities were more likely to show dysregulated DMN thought patterns such as catastrophizing, meaning that their thoughts were occupied with the sense that bad things can and will happen. In this case it might be recurring thoughts and worries that another disaster is imminent.

The participants who were more likely to catastrophize (dysregulated DMN thinking) showed more disturbances in felt experience. The high catastrophizers were less able to identify and regulate their emotions compared to low catastrophizers, who were more able to accept and feel the emotional challenges of what happened. People who were high on catastrophizing were also more likely to be diagnosed with symptoms of PTSD.[70] This type of research shows how thinking, feeling, and physical symptoms of PTSD can combine into a "package" or synergistic state of dysregulated ESA.

Dysregulated Autonomic Nervous System

Stress, trauma, and illness are at the heart of all forms of dysregulation, especially when a person has a life history of abuse and maltreatment, neglect, medical conditions and associated traumatic effects of treatment (chemotherapy, surgery, life support, implanted medical devices, etc.), war and being a refugee, accidents and injuries, loss of a parent, child, or spouse, being a member of a minority group facing the daily trauma of discrimination and hatred, and so on.[71] As we just saw, amygdala activation during stress alters the DMN thought network as it shuts down the modulating functions of the dorsomedial prefrontal cortex.

Similarly, the amygdala alters the function of the ventromedial prefrontal cortex, the regulatory part of the felt experience neural networks (Figure 2.3, p. 62). This means that when we are susceptible to stress (i.e., less resilient), have suffered a trauma (either from childhood or later life events such as war, assault, accidents, forced displacement, discrimination, and so on), or are prone to anxiety or depression, the amygdala becomes more activated while the DMN and felt experience networks become dysregulated.[72] The same amygdala activation that dysregulates thought and feeling also dysregulates the autonomic nervous system (ANS).[73]

The amygdala is massively linked to both the hypothalamic and brainstem centers of the ANS. The nervous system's appraisal of safety vs. threat—via the amygdala—can directly turn on and off sympathetic and parasympathetic pathways (including the vagal) and their corresponding stress hormones that directly affect our physiology, which makes us less resilient to even everyday stressors.

During states of dysregulated ESA, there is a hyperactivation of the sympathetic and/or (fearful dorsal vagal) parasympathetic nervous system resulting from current or prior unresolved threat, stress, or trauma. This means that we are either stuck "on" in an unrelenting state of high sympathetic arousal, accompanied by high levels of cortisol in the bloodstream, or we are stuck "off" in dorsal vagal shutdown and dissociation.

Being stuck sympathetically "on" means that we are continually in a fight-or-flight mode. We are spending most of our metabolic resources defending ourselves against or escaping from our uncomfortable felt experiences or real external threats in the current environment (an abusive spouse or parent, a dangerous neighborhood, racial and gender discrimination, being in a war zone, facing the dangers of being a refugee with an uncertain future), perceived threats (catastrophizing worry and anxiety about any of these conditions, generalized anxiety about social, family, or work situations), or past threats whose residues still infect our nervous system.

Unlike modulated ESA where we have some access to parasympathetic moments of settling and resetting our nervous system, in dysregulated ESA there is no ventral vagal or non-fear dorsal vagal parasympathetic activation and therefore no opportunity for rest, insight, discovery, problem solving, grounding, and so forth. In modulated ESA we may feel that we are pushing ourselves beyond our limits, but we still have the ability to regulate—that is, to slow down briefly and re-ground ourselves and our intentions. When dysregulated, we do not have that ability, and we suffer for that.

If we reframe dysregulated felt experience and thought from the perspective of the ANS, being in hypersympathetic stuck-on *fight* mode would include frustration, slow-burn anger or hostility, vigilance, watchfulness, muscle tension, high arousal, risky behavior from pushing limits and boundaries, tension in whole-body posture or expression, strained breathing, chronic pain, discomfort, and fatigue. In hypersympathetic stuck-on *flight* mode we would be avoiding, withdrawing, hiding, shrinking, making ourselves small or unnoticed, or self-harming; we would feel worthlessness, doubt, shame, an inability to "land" or settle, the urgency to move, anxiety, despair, or suicidal thoughts.

These states of the ANS are often accompanied by impaired forms of autonomic felt experience. Examples include uncontrollable and intense feelings such as heart racing, shortness of breath or rapid hyperventilation breathing, sweating, fidgeting and restlessness, dry mouth, dizziness, headaches, nausea, and digestive unrest.[74]

We can also be stuck off in dorsal vagal *freeze*. These are states of dissociation such as confusion, numbness, losing a train of thought, fatigue, depression, giving up, loss of self and initiative, "not there," vacantly gazing, dead inside, detachment, and lifelessness. We may also suffer from inattentiveness, distracted mind-wandering, and forgetfulness.[75] In extreme cases of dissociation, people can be diagnosed with depersonalization disorder, meaning they feel as if they are living outside of themselves, as if they are observing themselves from a distance. Not surprisingly, depersonalization disorder is also associated with an inability to accurately sense one's own emotional state.[76]

Some people believe that worry is good for them, a way to work out their problems. They seem to think that dysregulated DMN worries provide a similar review function as modulated DMN thinking. Researchers from the Universities of Cassino and Messina (Italy) reviewed thirty-one studies on worry that met multiple standards of high-quality scientific principles. It turned out that, across these studies, this belief in the importance of worry was detrimental to people's health. Worriers were more likely to suffer from depression, anxiety, and chronic health conditions.[77] Similar studies done at Florida State University (Tallahassee, USA) and at health centers in New Mexico and Texas (USA) show that ruminative worry impairs the ability to handle emotional distress and makes it more likely that worriers will turn to substance abuse or self-harming rather than more modulated strategies for self-calming.[78]

Summary and Conclusions

The research findings reviewed in this chapter suggest that in each of the three states of ESA, there is a synergistic relationship between felt experience, thoughts, and ANS activation. *Synergy* means that all these facets work together and influence each other in a self-sustaining feedback system; particular kinds of thoughts are most likely to co-occur with particular kinds of felt experience and particular forms of autonomic arousal.[79]

As mentioned in the previous section, for example, dysregulated thoughts like worries are partly evoked by a sense of threat in the ANS that destabilizes DMN thought. At the same time, the presence in our body of dysregulated worrisome thought patterns becomes a source of internal stress. We are stuck in these unproductive thought loops, and we can't make them stop. So distressed thinking feeds back into the stress detection network, via the amygdala, and further propels the ANS into states of being stuck on or stuck off.

The same kinds of feedback loops happen when we are stuck in the felt experience of pain, discomfort, anxiety, or depression. The body interprets these feelings as an emergency, which dysregulates the ANS. The dysregulated ANS (the sense that we cannot control our hyperarousal) feeds back to amplify the pain experience. For dysregulation, the synergy is an ongoing state of mutually cocreated autonomic hyperarousal, pain, disease states, and distressing thoughts.

In restorative states, on the other hand, feelings of calm and relaxation are so compelling that they support and amplify the continued activation of the parasympathetic nervous system. In states of modulated ESA, on- and off-task productive thinking carries with it a kind of momentum that keeps us sympathetically aroused. We get "hooked" on being engaged and productive or continuing to work until we figure something out that had been eluding a solution. We can still find moments of felt experience, but we get pulled by the sympathetic momentum back to the task.

Synergy does *not* mean that the ANS, felt experience, or thinking "controls" any of the others. Many healing practices, to be reviewed in the last chapter, make the assumption that our unproductive worries and anxious emotions, for example, "cause" ill health in the body. This assumption of causation leads to the conclusion that if we could just change how we think or if we were able to "release" the stuck emotions, then our body would be able to function in a more healthy manner.

These healing practices that start from a single component of the system (changing our thoughts, releasing our emotions, becoming more mindful, or shifting our "energy," for example) can sometimes be effective, at least for a short period of time. Since each state is a synergy, however, making a more permanent shift out of dysregulated states into modulated or restorative states is less likely to occur by simply shifting a single component (see the discussion earlier in this chapter about the limits of emotional intelligence).

Synergy means that all the pieces that compose a state of ESA are contributing to maintaining us in that state. For a more complete healing, we need to shift the whole synergistic system of, for example, dysregulated states. And we need to be able to sustain modulated states in a healthy manner and drop into restorative states in such a way that they last sufficiently long to bring a more healing experience.

The next chapters are about shifting between states. State changes are propelled by our embodied self-awareness of the entire synergy of what it feels like to be in restorative, modulated, or dysregulated ESA. Part of embodied self-awareness must therefore include learning to be honest with ourselves about the state in which our body is functioning at any given moment. The goal is to develop and refine our consciousness of our ESA states so that we can name and notice when, if, how, and under what circumstances we might shift into or remain in any one of the three states of ESA.

We have to learn to be honest with ourselves and accept that everyone, including us, gets dysregulated. Similarly, we all can find times when we are feeling modulated. Finding restorative states is more rare, but most of us are capable of feeling them when they happen. This practice of refining, naming, feeling, and accepting all our embodied states—and the shifts between them—is the first step toward transforming stuck dysregulated states into more productive and healthy modulated and restorative states.

Simply bringing nonjudgmental awareness to ourselves allows us to take action, find resources—such as medical interventions, psychotherapy, or complementary and alternative practices—and to have the self-confidence to know and trust ourselves from the inside out about the health care choices we make for ourselves.[80]

ESA—and restorative ESA in particular—is a real neurophysiological function of the body, equally important as the organic functions of our cardiovascular, respiratory, or digestive system. Awareness of our embodied state activates a real cellular process of maintaining and monitoring health across multiple body functional systems. The challenge is that becoming self-aware is much more difficult in practice than these words might imply.

Under conditions of illness, stress, and trauma, which affect almost every human on the planet, our nervous system is remarkably good at hiding us from ourselves. The truth is that we cannot cultivate this nonjudgmental embodied self-awareness on our own. We need the support of a loved one, or a trusted guide and facilitator, one whose work is dedicated not to teaching us a practice or technique but helping us simply feel the blind spots in our own ESA experiences.

In the next chapters, you will find an open invitation to sense and feel, to accept yourself as you are, to recognize our common humanity with its possibilities and frailties. You may be surprised, or discouraged, or enlivened. You will certainly be changed from the person who you may think you are into a closer relationship to the person who is more truly yourself.

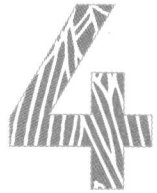

The Felt Experience of Maintaining or Changing States of Embodied Self-Awareness

Embodied self-awareness (ESA) is our experience of the inner condition of the body, our awareness of how we think and feel about ourselves in any given moment in each of the three states: restorative, modulated, or dysregulated. This chapter is about learning how to discern when we are in any given state of ESA and also when and how we shift between the states.

We all need time in restorative parasympathetic states in order for our body's functional systems to recover from their daily and long-term traumatic stressors. Being in a beautiful spot in the natural world, for example, can create a sense of awe. That sense can be momentary, a brief distraction from our conversation with a companion or a stream of thought. This is what happens in modulated ESA.

But even if we are primarily in a "doing" mode of being modulated, we have the opportunity to notice this brief moment as a possible gateway into a restorative state of ESA. We could, at this particular moment in time, choose to let ourselves be fully present with the awe, to "sink into" it and let it take us to a deeper state of relaxation.

For that to happen, for us to shift from modulated to restorative ESA, we have to make a conscious choice to let go of thoughts or conversations in modulated ESA and just be here now in restorative ESA. This choice, based on the awareness of the possibility that we could really give ourselves the gift of shifting into a restorative state, is an inner invitation into prolonged parasympathetic relief.

Ideally, if we are aware of the possibility and power of restorative states, we can use our ESA to feel them emerging. Our cue might be modulated thoughts like: "Wow! This place is so amazing! I just want to be here and take it in—watch the clouds pass or the waves tumble, or be transfixed by the starlight—and make that choice to open up to what is there around me."

The pull of living inside modulated states is so compelling, however, that it may not feel right or safe or natural to let go of our TPN (task-positive net-work) and DMN (default-mode network) thoughts. We can get enchanted with our own inner poetry or with staying connected to our conversational partner. So we just keep going: walking past the beauty, or convincing our-selves that we are content to continue these mental or interpersonal dia-logues. This going and going—this enchantment of being so beautifully modulated—has its limits. If we continue with this kind of mental sympa-thetic engagement, at some point our body systems will start to break down and lead us into dysregulation and possible health crises.

This chapter will help you become better attuned to how each state feels. It will also help you to sense the "momentum" or "pull" of each state once you have landed in it. Finally, this chapter will offer some clues about how to break out of unproductive, or productive but draining, states and aim for something that feels more restorative.

Dysregulated ESA, for example, is a stuck state that most often requires us to seek help in order to find our way into modulated functioning. We may not be able to free ourselves from the entrapment of dysregulation. That's just the truth. What we can do for ourselves, however, is to honestly confess to ourselves, or to someone we trust, that we are caught and need help. To do that, we need to cultivate our awareness of how it feels to be dysregulated. That little bit of modulated awareness, even in the throes of being dysregulated, gives us a tiny opportunity to find the support we need to regain our ability to better self-modulate: to begin the shift out of dysregulation.

To make the shift from dysregulation to modulation, or from modulated to restorative states, means that we need to have a sense that there is a better way to live and to feel. So the choice to seek help when dysregulated requires multiple kinds of self-awareness: that we are, in this moment, dysregulated; that we are aware of what living in a modulated or a restorative state feels like; and that we are also aware that there are people, practices, or care providers that are useful in shifting our state of ESA.

The premise of this book is that our awareness of all these forms of embodied self-awareness is essential in maintaining health and recovery from illness. Our embodied self-awareness of all three states, and of how it feels when we change from one state into another, is to be in possession of a map of the territory of our inner experience. This awareness gives us an onboard GPS of where we are located at any moment and also, on the map, the routes we need to take to arrive at the other locations (states of ESA) in the landscape of embodied consciousness. Moving around this territory and noticing the thoughts and feelings that occur in each location—and along the routes between locations—create the possibility that we can shift into more productive and healing states of being.[1]

The Neurophysiology of Switching between States of Embodied Self-Awareness

Restorative ESA, as described in chapters 2 and 3, is clearly an optimal state of being. There is nothing else like it. In restorative ESA we are transformed and taken outside of our usual self into realms of peace, comfort, rest, and even transcendence. Why not just stay there? What would make us move into modulated or dysregulated ESA? Or if we are in one of these other two states, how can we get back to a more restorative state?

The area of the nervous system that is responsible for allowing us to remain in one state of ESA, or to shift from one to another, is the medial prefrontal cortex.[2] As shown in Figures 1.5 (p. 21) and 2.1 (p. 52), the medial prefrontal cortex is divided between dorsal (toward the top of the head) and ventral (toward the base of the head) portions.

The dorsomedial prefrontal cortex helps keep up our DMN thoughts, those we have about the self and others when we are off-task—in a creative, imaginative mode. When the amygdala detects stress, it suppresses the regulating functions of the dorsomedial prefrontal cortex on DMN thoughts. These thoughts become dysregulated: ruminative, self-absorbed, anxious, and self-centered.[3]

The ventromedial prefrontal cortex has a similar function for felt experience. Under conditions of safety and low stress, the ventromedial prefrontal cortex helps sustain felt experience and suppress TPN and DMN thoughts in a way that leads to rest, relaxation, relief, and restoration of all the body systems.[4]

The ventromedial prefrontal cortex also plays an important role in the formation of emotionally significant memories.[5] These might include positive memories such as moments of generosity or love, or negative memories such as incidents of feeling shame or rejection. In general, circumstances in the past or the present that are the most emotionally self-relevant will be associated with higher activation of the ventromedial prefrontal cortex.[6] Under conditions of challenge, illness, stress, and trauma—both modulated and dysregulated—activity in the ventromedial prefrontal cortex becomes suppressed, and felt experience becomes diminished and brief.[7]

One study on the ventromedial prefrontal cortex was done by researchers at the University of Texas at Austin (USA) and the University of California, Los Angeles (USA). They found that increased risk taking decreased activation in the ventromedial prefrontal cortex. Using a method called the Balloon Analog Risk Task, participants were trained to inflate simulated balloons shown on a computer monitor. They could get monetary rewards for each successive "pump" of the balloon, and they could do as many pumps as they wanted during a fixed time period. The participants could choose to "cash out" at any point during this time period and save their winnings.

But the simulated balloon might explode during this time period. If this happened, participants would lose all the money accumulated during that period. They could, however, keep any money earned in prior periods if the balloon did not explode. Thus, each new pump of the balloon constituted a risk of losing at least some of their earned reward. The results showed that the activation of the ventromedial prefrontal cortex decreased in direct proportion to the growing size of the balloon.[8]

This is a simple and elegant demonstration of the inverse relationship between stress/risk level and the ability of the ventromedial prefrontal cortex to maintain felt experience. Put another way, as the risk of the balloon exploding increased, participants were less able to access their own felt experience. Maybe tuning out of our felt experience is an adaptive strategy when we are faced with risky situations, a way to get through a difficult challenge? Or, conversely, maybe we indulge in risky activities because we want to avoid facing what we are feeling?

During modulated states, the dorsomedial prefrontal cortex takes over the regulatory role from the ventromedial prefrontal cortex. This means that modulated thinking via the TPN and DMN becomes the salient mode of experience as feelings are relatively suppressed.[9] During dysregulated states, both of these branches of the medial prefrontal cortex go off-line, leaving us without access to modulatory strategies and therefore prey to unpleasant felt experiences such as pain and muscle tension and intrusive thoughts such as worry and self-blame.[10] People who have prefrontal brain injuries, or damage to the prefrontal cortex from dementia or Alzheimer's, have reduced or absent self-awareness in some or all of the domains of felt experience and thought.[11]

Besides the medial prefrontal cortex, other areas of the prefrontal cortex also play a role in supporting the modulation of thinking and feeling. The dorso*lateral* prefrontal cortex (see Figure 1.3, p. 15) helps with the modulation of productive thought—focusing attention on a problem or issue—using the TPN.

The orbitofrontal cortex (see Figure 2.5, p. 68) provides the ability to discern the emotional value of experience.[12] Recall from chapter 2 that emotional value is the feeling of wanting to approach or avoid, to have more or less of something. This prefrontal evaluation aspect of emotion works together with the insula for feeling emotional states, and with the anterior cingulate cortex and sensorimotor cortices to provide the motivational component of emotion: the creation of body expressions and movements related to getting closer or farther away.

During states of dysregulated ESA, it is difficult to discern our emotional state, meaning that there is a suppression of the normal function of the orbitofrontal cortex. If we can't discern if something is good or bad for us, helpful or harmful, we are destined to feel lost and disoriented. The more people suppress emotional evaluation, the more likely it is that they will sink into the mire of dysregulated ruminations and fears.[13]

Productive thought becomes replaced by confusion and rumination without the modulatory effects of the prefrontal cortex.[14] Our ability to be creative, solve problems, make plans, respond to novel situations, sense our emotions, and modify our behavior to fit the current situation all become compromised with illness, stress, and trauma and their suppressive effects on prefrontal function.[15] When the amygdala and hypothalamus are sensing threat, stress, or trauma, we shift away from rest or productivity into putting all the systems of the body into survival mode (fight, flight, freeze).

In summary, the process of becoming aware of and shifting between states of ESA is related to the functioning of the prefrontal cortex. As we practice and cultivate the ability to shift out of stressful and traumatic dysregulated states and into states of modulated and restorative ESA, therefore, we are strengthening our prefrontal neural networks, building connections and neural pathways in the same way that we build muscle tissue with physical exercise. In this chapter, you will find ways to exercise your prefrontal networks so that you may increase the likelihood of maintaining yourself in modulated and restorative states of ESA.

The Journey out of Dysregulated and into Modulated Embodied Self-Awareness

Dysregulated ESA is a stuck state. Dysregulated means that we do not have volitional control over what we experience; we are enslaved to unproductive, unhealthy, and dangerous feelings and actions. It means that we cannot escape from prolonged states of dysregulated ESA on our own. If we could, then we would be capable of sustaining a state of modulated ESA. We usually need the help of other people to break out of the stuckness of dysregulation.

Not all people who are dysregulated are willing to do this. Part of dysregulation is the sense of not needing and not wanting help. The self-centeredness of some types of dysregulation blinds people to the ways in which their actions are self-destructive, to the harm they cause others, and to the havoc they create in their families, communities, and workplaces.

Most people in a dysregulated state are victims of trauma, much of which has its origins in early life history. It begins with abusive or neglectful parenting, dangerous neighborhoods, bullying and shunning at school, poverty, war, environmental disasters (floods, earthquakes, fires), discrimination against and persecution of groups of people because of their gender, culture, or skin color, and living as a child refugee with no homeland.

Early- and later-life trauma can also come from illnesses such as cancer and its treatment, disabilities, and subsequent surgeries and prosthetics; birth defects; mental and cognitive impairments; stigmatization from being under- or overweight; skin color or physical appearance; and poverty and disadvantage. In the time period in which this book is being written, people are suffering from one of the worst plagues in recorded human history. This, along with the effects of rapidly accelerating climate change and economic hardship, is already creating an environment in which dysregulated states are becoming more common.

A team of researchers from the University of Melbourne and Monash University (Australia) and the medical school at Harvard University (Boston, Massachusetts, USA) concluded that:

> The prevalence of symptoms of anxiety disorder in June 2020 was approximately three times those reported in the second quarter of 2019 (25.5% versus 8.1%) … depressive disorder was approximately four times that reported in the second quarter of 2019 (24.3% versus 6.5%) … Suicidal ideation was also elevated; approximately twice as many respondents reported serious consideration of suicide in the previous 30 days than did adults in the United States in 2018, referring to the previous 12 months (10.7% versus 4.3%).[16]

We like to think of trauma as arising from a specific catastrophic event, but the fact is that trauma—a dysregulated disturbance of the nervous system—is perversely ordinary, something that happens to just about everyone. According to psychologist Mark Epstein, author of the book *The Trauma of Everyday Life*,

> *Trauma is not just the result of major disasters. It does not happen to only some people. An undercurrent of trauma runs through ordinary life ... One way or another, death (and its cousins: old age, illness, accidents, separation and loss) hangs over all of us. Nobody is immune. Our world is unstable and unpredictable, and operates, to a great degree and despite incredible scientific advancement, outside our ability to control it.* [17]

Crime, racism, sexism, other forms of discrimination and inequality, the pandemic, climate change, serious illnesses, and family disruption due to divorce, death, and domestic violence are, unfortunately, part of everyday life; few escape unaffected. Thankfully, most health care professionals now know how trauma affects the body, memory, behavior, sense of self, and felt experience via dysregulation of the autonomic nervous system. [18]

The first step out of dysregulated ESA is to become more aware of how this state feels in the moment. This awareness of being dysregulated is facilitated when people understand that dysregulation is a "normal" or expected part of the human condition when the body is under stress or has suffered trauma. [19]

We have to sense and admit that we are stuck, hurt, immobilized, or in self-destructive patterns. Yes, coming to that realization can be horrible. The feeling is that we will never escape this state, that we will continue to suffer, that there is no way out. Yet the miracle of embodied self-awareness is that this honest self-realization is actually a ticket out of dysregulation. You don't yet know how, you don't yet have the resources, but by this simple awareness of your condition, you have initiated a change process into modulated thinking about your dysregulation.

Part of the felt experience of being dysregulated is the sense of "too much" feeling: too much pain, too much fatigue, too much sadness, too much intensity and inability to slow down, too much uncontrollable rage. Dysregulation feels unbearable.

One reason we are stuck in fight, flight, and freeze responses is that these intense, "too much" feelings trigger the amygdala to sense that we are in danger. In this case, the danger is coming from inside our body, from our own thoughts and feelings. It does not matter that the external sources of danger and trauma may have occurred many years ago. Anything that reminds us of the trauma sets off all the survival mechanisms. (The memories of emotionally salient events are encoded in the hippocampus, which is directly adjacent to the amygdala.)

This survival coping strategy helps push away overwhelming feelings and thoughts in a process of "experiential avoidance." According to Steven C. Hayes, a professor of psychology at the University of Nevada who has received awards for his research on experiential avoidance and has given much-viewed TED talks, this avoidance consists of being "unwilling to remain in contact with particular private experiences (e.g., bodily sensations, emotions, thoughts, memories, behavioral predispositions) and [taking] steps to alter the form or frequency of these events and the content that occasion them."[20]

We are no longer escaping, fighting, or freezing from the original danger: we are doing these things to help us escape this sense of "too much" that is coming from inside our own body. The fact is, because we have avoided these feelings for sometimes many years, we don't really know if what we are trying to avoid feeling will, in fact, be too much for us to handle.

Our felt experience of our bodily sensations, emotions, and thoughts is triggering in the insula a fearful interpretation of what these feelings *might be like*. Felt experience is already "fuzzy" because of unmyelinated pathways between the peripheral and central nervous systems that make it hard for the insula to locate the source and content of the feeling. Our prior traumatic history with intense felt experience adds another layer of fuzzy uncertainty. Because our body shifts so quickly into dysregulated defensive strategies for experiential avoidance, the only embodied interpretation of felt experience with which we are familiar is that it is dangerous.[21]

When things feel "too much," not only are we likely to avoid the experience within ourselves, but we also have the tendency to shift attention away from ourselves, as when we channel our own unbearable feelings in the form of anger at others. Dysregulated anger and hostility usually come from an inability to grasp, feel, and accept one's own feelings of traumatic abandonment, abuse, loss, or whatever.

These underlying and unfelt feelings are the true self, which remains hidden from us because these feelings come from something painful, unresolved, and unrecognized, something that happened to us in our past. Moving out of dysregulated ESA and into modulated ESA is a process of becoming more present with our felt experiences and unwanted thoughts. It is a process in which we move beyond experiential avoidance and settle into ourselves, so that we have the possibility to bypass the feeling of "too much."

With the right kind of guidance, it is indeed possible to learn to bear these intense feelings. It is certainly possible to do this alone, but for most of us, the pathway out of dysregulation is interpersonal. We need to feel safe enough and sufficiently confident in another trusted person in order to move past our habitual fight, flight, and freeze patterns of responding.

At first, we learn to stay more in the present moment, even for brief periods of time, with this simple awareness: that up until now, many of our experiences felt like too much. Getting familiar with the feeling that our inner experience may be unbearable is, in fact, an emerging state of modulated ESA. This starting point is often enough to begin a developmental transition from living primarily in states of dysregulated ESA into being able to consistently maintain states of modulated ESA.

To take one example, suppose you are wearing a mask to protect against COVID or air pollution, and you begin to feel shortness of breath and an emerging sense of panic. Now, in actuality, you *can* breathe. You might have to take some deeper breaths, and you might have to convince yourself that you are, in this moment, OK and safe. Nevertheless, the current situation is triggering a psychophysiological response that may be set off by a memory of a past experience of being in some real danger, or of once having a heart or asthma attack, or of having been in an ICU with respiratory distress and needing a breathing tube.

The felt experience, the interoception of shortness of breath right now, is intertwined in our neural circuitry with a traumatic memory, leading to an embodied interpretation or inference that we are still in danger. Our embodied self may "know" in thought that we are really OK, but our physiology is pushing us into an interpretation of the present-moment interoception that the shortness of breath is a prelude to panic.

Sometimes we simply can't prevent the onset of a panic attack when we are in the middle of, for example, crossing the street, or in a work meeting, or even in an intimate setting. What we can do, however, is notice which situations are most likely to trigger such an attack. The more we become familiar with how our current and prior life history and trauma experiences push us into dysregulated states, therefore, the more likely we are to be able to name and accept "what is": that when we feel short of breath, we automatically begin to sink into dysregulation.

Telling about our experience to another person, such as a close companion or a trained embodied therapist, can help us "get" how our body might have come up with a mistaken interoceptive inference of danger (we got scared, the situation reminded us of a prior fearful event) even when that situation is not overtly dangerous. This type of TPN reasoning, facilitated by someone who really "hears" our story, is an important component in building a more modulated state of ESA.[22]

It may feel supportive to learn that our habitual dysregulated response is perfectly normal. It may, for some of us, help to understand in TPN thought how our own personal history of trauma may have contributed to the way in which a relatively innocuous recent experience may have become converted into a state of dysregulation. Thinking and explaining are useful aspects of modulated ESA, especially when we are in the early phases of "growing" our ability to feel more clearly the shortness of breath, or any discomfort, pain, anger, sadness, loss, or whatever is present that, in the past, felt like "too much."

Acceptance of our ways of becoming dysregulated is, therefore, a key factor in growing our awareness in a way that leads to a shift into more modulated states. *Acceptance does not mean that the patterns of dysregulation are an acceptable way to live, nor does it mean that the prior life experiences and trauma that may have contributed to the current dysregulation are acceptable or even forgivable.* Acceptance means that in this present moment, we are growing our ability to simply acknowledge how we get thrown off, the ways we get overwhelmed, or our typical pathways into not being able to control our thoughts, feelings, or actions.[23]

TAKE A BREAK

Suppose you are wanting to take a break from some demanding task, and you decide to make yourself a cup of coffee. This, you might be thinking, would be a good way to modulate the potential dysregulation of the possibly compulsive demands of that task.

You go to the kitchen—at home or at work or wherever—thinking hopefully about sitting and enjoying your nice drink. When you arrive, however, you see that the coffee pot has not been cleaned by the previous user. As you are emptying the grounds and washing the filter and pot, you go to reach for the coffee canister and find that it is empty or nearly so. So then you have to go digging in the cabinets. Maybe there is no more coffee, maybe the sugar and cream are low, maybe you need to start a shopping list.

You finally get everything together, and by this time you are definitely annoyed. Perhaps you don't want the coffee anymore, and you are thinking about finding the person who left the mess and left the pantry empty. You are thinking about making sure they know how pissed off they made you feel. Most likely, however, you just keep pushing ahead with following the steps of making the coffee, getting more tense and more aggravated all the while.

You wanted to make the coffee because you were slipping into a dysregulated loop of overworking, and now you are caught in another loop in which you are even more dysregulated. You have to keep going; you have to finish this simple, stupid, ridiculous little task of making the damn coffee!

Can you modulate by slowing yourself down? Can you take this in stride and see all the extra steps as just a part of the break, which is now actually being extended so you don't have to go right back to work? Or, do you push yourself and let your ruminations take over? Do you start to make little mistakes (too much water, or too little coffee, or spilling water on the counter while filling the reservoir)? OK, you can feel yourself getting dysregulated but, hey, you are almost done, you are almost there. A few more steps and you'll have your coffee.

But did you notice that you were getting tired? That your stress level was rising? That you couldn't break the seemingly compelling chain of this step, then the next step, and then the next one that was pushing you forward? Maybe if you had noticed the rising sympathetic activation, you could have stopped yourself and taken a real break from all the task-oriented doing. Maybe you could have asked for help? Maybe there is a nearby café to which you could take a nice walk and get out of the building? Maybe...

To take a real break—one that gives space for at least a few moments of parasympathetic downtime—is a process of accepting our level of stress, irritation, and negative thoughts. *We also have to admit to ourselves that this psychophysiological reaction is coming from inside of ourself, our out-of-control nervous system,* and that our reaction is objectively out of proportion to the current circumstances. This awareness is often sufficient to initiate a momentary pause where we can actually envision a concrete possibility to slow down, feel, and accept how we can get easily dysregulated, and thus make a real shift into modulated ESA.

Particularly with a history of trauma inflicted upon us by other people, we may come to believe that we are bad, wrong, unwanted, not worthy, not good enough, or shameful. These feelings of negative self-worth go along with the sense of being out of control and "too much," or as in the sidebar, the feeling that we have to do it all ourselves, and if we can't it's a personal failure.

Part of acceptance is grasping that what happened in that past traumatic situation is not our fault and that we have a right and responsibility to define ourselves in a new way that better fits the person we are now or the person we would like to become.[24] We can say no to getting worked up and yes to really embracing that break: we can transform stress into eustress.

Over time, as we are more able to stay in the present moment in modulated states of ESA, the thoughts and feelings underneath the dysregulated feelings—the ones connected to the original trauma—can begin to emerge in awareness. These may be feelings of abandonment, betrayal, shame, loss, fear, justifiable anger, sadness, and grief along with the thoughts of being unworthy.[25]

Shifting into a state of modulated ESA means that these feelings may begin to occur at least briefly and we can have modulated thoughts about them: "Yes, I am really annoyed. I wish I wasn't so hard on myself. I gotta stop and breathe or this job is going to kill me. It's time to have a talk with my (spouse, boss, partner, parent, child, friend)." The key to unlocking dysregulation's hold on our thoughts and feelings is first to be able to notice and name the times, places, and ways in which we tend to get dysregulated in our present life. The experience of dysregulation is different for every person.

We may, for example, experience moments of time when we lose touch with both our thoughts and our feelings, a form of dysregulation known as *dissociation*. Everyone gets dissociated from time to time. It's normal. If we don't feel well, if we are distracted or can't focus our thoughts, if we are "on" all the time rushing around and nonstop busy, we are experiencing mild-to-moderate forms of dissociation from our felt experience and modulated thoughts.

For some people, dissociation shows up as mental confusion, like a brain fog. Some people forget ordinary things, like the day of the week or where they left their keys or wallet. Some people space out and lose track of a conversation or get lost in the middle of a task. Sometimes we discover a bruise or sore spot and don't remember how the injury happened. More serious forms of dissociation show up when people actively suppress their thoughts or felt experiences by using substances, self-harming, pushing beyond their limits, or taking risks to blot out pain and discomfort. Noticing how and when we dissociate—or have any other form of dysregulated felt experiences or thinking—is key to beginning a shift out of dysregulated ESA into states of modulated ESA where we can catch glimpses of long-hidden feelings. As we are learning to be able to modulate our felt experience—by using TPN and DMN emotional intelligence strategies, for example—there may be a desire to speed up the process of recovery. If we can feel a little bit of the shame at first, then why not just feel it all? Well, for one, it is impossible to suddenly jump from long-term suppression of felt experience into a deep feeling of shame or hurt because our autonomic nervous system has spent years developing pathways to avoid those difficult feelings; in our past, it was not safe to feel them.

I conducted a research study with three ESA practitioners doing Rosen Method bodywork. Each practitioner in this study had at least twenty years of clinical experience. Two of them worked with two different clients and one of them with one client, for a total of five clients, and each client was seen for sixteen sessions.

Following each bodywork session, the practitioners wrote for one hour about the important events in the session in the sequence in which these events occurred, rather than simply writing a summary of the session. Reading through these post-session notes, I was easily able to classify over 90 percent of the practitioners' statements into one the three ESA states: restorative, modulated, or dysregulated. And because the session notes were written in chronological order, I could see the sequence in which events occurred during the session.

This resulting division of each session into a sequence of ESA states allowed for the possibility to study how states shifted from one to another. *The data revealed that there were no instances—none at all—in which a state of dysregulated ESA shifted directly into a state of restorative ESA.* Rather, clients either stayed in the same state of ESA, or if they did shift states, it was between dysregulated and modulated ESA, or else between modulated and restorative ESA.[26]

This means that if we have been primarily dysregulated, we must first learn to access and maintain a state of modulated ESA before we can "graduate" into restorative ESA. It also means that modulated ESA is a transitional state that always occurs in between states of dysregulated and restorative ESA. Modulated ESA, therefore, is an essential first step out of being dysregulated.

Knowing that leaping from dysregulation into restoration is just not going to happen, we can use our growing ability to access modulated thinking to let ourselves accept that it is enough at first to feel and own little bits and pieces of dysregulated felt experience. *A small amount of felt experience in modulated states of ESA is, in fact, the only route out of dysregulated ESA.* Sorry, but this journey out of dysregulation is a local bus or train route with lots of stops along the way: no express line is available!

Being able to modulate the intensity of trauma and pain by breaking it into small bits is a gift, really, a way of protecting ourselves from becoming overwhelmed or even retraumatized. It's healthy and productive to be patient with ourselves and to cultivate small doses of felt experience in a modulated way. We feel a little bit, then we try to make sense of the feeling or the memory of where it came from. Using our TPN and DMN thinking in this way can be extremely helpful in stabilizing and regulating the felt experience, so we can understand and metabolize it before it becomes "too much."

Recovering from a lifetime of suppression, dissociation, and trauma is similar to recovering from a serious illness—a bad case of the flu, a broken bone, a surgery, or a chronic illness like cancer or cardiovascular disease. We don't just jump out of bed one day and come back into full health. It may take days or weeks or even years to recover our full strength and well-being. We have to accept that healing takes the time it needs, and the best thing we can do to facilitate that healing is to respect the limits of our cellular embodiment.

Another aspect of getting more grounded into modulated states is the possibility of making choices based on what we actually want rather than choosing what we have been told to want. This can be simple, at least at first. It might be choosing clothing that makes us feel good and that comes from our own values related to, say, comfort or our ability to move in certain ways, or wearing colors that we love but we came to think were forbidden, or wearing clothes that fit our gender, cultural, or racial identity. In this process, we are redefining ourselves, and it can be a wonderful journey into self-discovery.[27]

We can later graduate to more advanced self-clarifying choices such as how we express our ideas to other people, explain our preferences and desires for sexual gratification and expression, or alter our sexual or gender identity. Each of these important life choices and decisions may take months or years and require a good deal of conscious self-modulation: solving personal issues of identity using our TPN or reflecting on how other people respond to us using our DMN. In this phase, we are able to access feelings but in a modulated way—that is, briefly and as a source of useful information to help in the modulation process.

Recovery from dysregulation requires this essential ability to self-modulate, to reclaim our body and define our identity and desires. We saw from the research study on Rosen Method bodywork that people don't suddenly "arrive" in a restorative state directly from dysregulation, particularly if the dysregulation has gone on for long periods. There will be a lengthy process—possibly months or years—of shifting between dysregulation and modulation as the nervous system begins to change: as the window of tolerance/regulation of strong feelings opens, as trust in the safety of the setting and of our support systems begins to develop.[28]

During modulated ESA, people can also become aware of when they shift back into states of dysregulated ESA. This type of awareness, which was not available to us in the past, is an important part of regaining a more modulated state. The awareness of simply feeling ourselves moving into rumination or dissociation, for example, can awaken strategies for self-modulation. These strategies might include acceptance that we have a tendency to get dysregulated in a particular manner, in particular locations, or with particular people. This creates the possibility that we can actively reach out for help or guidance, or find resources in everyday life that help us return to a more modulated state.

The thesis of this book is that a full and productive life includes having regular and reliable access to states of restorative ESA. The take-home message of this section on the differences between dysregulated and modulated ESA, however, is that to move out of habitual, old, and traumatic patterns of dysregulation, we must first gain regular and reliable access to modulated ESA. Building resilience is like building muscle mass: it takes a lot of reps over a long time. For many people, the resilience of maintaining modulation is such an important achievement that it can feel like regaining control over their life, reestablishing safe and fulfilling relationships, and increasing a sense of well-being and health. Yes, more is possible, but for many people, being solidly and reliably modulated may be enough.

Shifting between Modulated and Restorative States of Embodied Self-Awareness

No matter how much the past may cast a shadow over the future, the very next phase of my ongoing way of being bodily is not unequivocally determined. There is room for transformation, be this a slight initial shift at the leading edge of the living present—a subtle sense of release somewhere in my body, for example—or a decisive moment of "deep change" reverberating in one way or another throughout my entire life.[29]

> —ELIZABETH BEHNKE, FROM AN ARTICLE PUBLISHED IN *THE HUMANISTIC PSYCHOLOGIST*, 2010. (She is a member of the Study Project in Phenomenology of the Body, a networking group founded in 1987.)

For any activity to be restorative—doing yoga or tai chi, meditating, listening to or dancing to or making music, going for a walk in nature, being intimate with another being, taking a bath (what activities lead to restorative states for you?)—there must be a felt parasympathetic response, a deepening into a sense of peace and mystery and oneness.

Going to parties and letting ourselves get wild and free, having engaging, deep, humorous, or intensely erotic encounters with other people, doing leaps on a skateboard, taking a run in the park: these are not restorative activities. They may be refreshing. They may be fulfilling. They may make us happy or excited. But they are all accompanied by sympathetic arousal; they take effort and modulation, thought and focused attention.

Restoration means that we have to let go of all of that doing, achieving, and hard-earned modulating control. This is extremely challenging. Most of us have devoted our lives and our personal healing paths to mastering challenges and gaining some degree of resilient self-control and self-regulation over previously dysregulated thinking and feeling.

Is it really possible, given that we may feel reasonably resilient in our ability to maintain modulated ESA, to simply relax and trust that whatever we are feeling is "right" in that present moment?[30] Is it possible to abandon those carefully worked-out thought schemes—making informed choices, noticing and managing our emotions using our emotional intelligence—that have been a fundamental part of holding us together and making sense of our way of being? Is it possible to set aside our well-practiced movement skills that make us artistic or athletic or romantic and give us a sense of self-worth and personal power?

Really, why would you want to just jump off a very stable, solid cliff into a huge sea of not-knowing? Why would you allow the flow of your feelings to take you on a very unpredictable ride down a series of emotional rapids and strong currents? The reward for letting go of our self-control is being able to enter the peace, grace, and healing of restorative states. Like jumping off that metaphorical cliff, you won't know what this experience is going to feel like until you try it because you can't plan it or understand it using your modulated thoughts, and you can't wear a life vest.

You can, however, be with someone who has done this before, someone who literally or metaphorically holds your hand and acts as your guide into the wilderness within yourself.

You won't be able to use your modulated thinking to get you into or help you stay in restorative ESA. If you have any thoughts—any mental tracking of what you are doing, any kind of planning or organizing your approach to being embodied, doing deliberate exercises to become embodied—then you are *not* in a restorative state. You are most likely firmly holding on to your modulated ESA. You only *think* you are in restorative ESA, which keeps you sympathetically aroused and prevents you from dropping into that ultimate experiential reward: a sustained parasympathetic state of relief and non-doing.

How can we support the shift from modulation to restoration? Letting go of modulated doing is a double-edged sword. From a modulated state of ESA, we can go either way: into the dysregulated collapse and dissociation of a fearful dorsal vagal state, or into a restorative, safe dorsal vagal state of deep rest and relaxation. According to Merete Holm Brantbjerg, a body psychotherapist from Denmark,

> *Nourishing the self is an activity, whether it is with food, contact, movement, nature, experiences or inspiration. It takes presence and bodily skills to let go of what one is doing, orient to what resources of nourishment are available, and choose, reach for, take*

in and digest them. How do we support presence when relaxing so we are capable of regenerating in exchange with the world around us instead of collapsing?[31]

Earlier we used the metaphor of a landscape of ESA and a roadmap for shifting between dysregulated and modulated states. That map is reasonably well defined. Unfortunately, the map is totally undefined and completely useless when we want to navigate from modulated to restorative states.

Since we don't have a map, here is a rough guide to what might happen. As we begin to let ourselves feel more, we might sense the outlines of an old pain or memory, a longing, or a sadness. We might remember, for example, how we had to work so hard as a child to please our parents, how we were always "on" yet never quite enough. We might remember our desire for love, hugs, and approval that never came and the exhaustion of our tiny body's resources as we struggled to earn that love.

If we continue to feel into ourselves and the felt experiences of childhood memories, maybe we will notice the muscle tension in our eyes, or neck, or arms, or belly: the places where we are exerting an unconscious but very physical form of self-control to keep working and thinking about how to get that love. This might lead us right back into the interpretation that these feelings are too much to handle, and a shift from modulated to dysregulated ESA.

In a modulated state, we can sense that these feelings are there inside of us, but they are in a kind of shadow, just outside of awareness. As we get closer to these feelings, we can become aware of something "larger" or more threatening, something deeper in the darkness beyond the shadow, something that we may be afraid to feel or confront. Out in the full light of awareness are our thoughts and worries. In the shadow, there is the edge of muscle tension, or physical or emotional pain, and maybe some sense of tears wanting to form in the corners of our eyes.

Yet it does not seem safe to go any further, at least not on our own, not without someone's support or guidance. Assuming that we don't sink back into dysregulation, we might succumb to an effortful attempt to modulate these feelings. To remain modulated, we fall back on our usual coping strategies like getting on with our lives, thinking about what needs next to be done, or even practicing yoga or meditation in a deliberate effort to soothe ourselves.

It is at this point, when we can develop an awareness of ourselves getting caught up in effortful modulation, that we have a choice. We can continue to cope by doing the modulated things we have come to rely on to keep ourselves under control. Or we can choose to find a way to move closer to a state of restorative ESA.

In the latter case, it is usually a good time, if the right person is available, for a phone or video call or asking for a hug of reassurance. This nonjudgmental social contact may be enough to allow the tears to come and the body to relax into a state that is coming closer to feeling restorative. Other people may be crucial for this step because we have to feel completely safe in order to willingly relax our entrenched modulated habits of holding on for dear life.

If we feel safe enough to let the "darker" feeling emerge, then we have to turn around and face these demons. We have to feel the constrictions in our breathing, in our chest, in our face. We have to feel how our tight diaphragm creates a constant sense of impending suffocation. We have to feel the distension in our gut from gas and bloating, or the heartburn in our chest, or the emerging discomfort in our pelvis. We have to be with the tickle in our throat and the urge to cough. We have to make contact with the deeper wells of sadness, fear, and anger.

To enter into the portal of restoration—as opposed to dropping into the experiential avoidance of dysregulation—is to allow ourselves to feel all (or any part) of this and not react, not try to make it better, not let the fear distract us from the felt experience of discomfort. The key to doing this is within the domain of modulated ESA.

During modulated ESA, we are mostly sympathetically aroused by the strategies we are using to remain in control. But there is a *potential space* where we can feel and settle into a tense muscle or held gut or moment of sadness for a few moments and notice that this can lead to a short but real feeling of ease.

We can "catch" a worry forming in our thoughts. Should we go to a social event where we might feel overwhelmed or not seen? Should we approach another person and say something that we have been meaning to tell them? Should we go out of our house when we don't feel safe (because of neighborhood dangers, or our skin color, or sexuality, or poverty, or even wealth and white privilege)?

Modulating means that we can "sit with" or "be with" the worry and think logically about the feelings that come up around it. Is the anticipated danger a real threat in our current environment, or are we plagued by a traumatic memory of a dangerous situation at an earlier point in our life? Or perhaps there is no such traumatic memory, but we are just feeling lonely, scared, or vulnerable.

As we use our TPN to "figure this out," we can create that potential space in modulated ESA to be with these feelings and see what else comes up for us in our thoughts or felt experiences. We can be observers of our own reactions and make thoughtful inferences. "When I let myself feel this fear (or anger, or pain), then I noticed that it wasn't as bad as I thought it might be." "When I allowed myself some space for opening up to a challenging feeling, I noticed that I felt safe with it for a while, but then my old defenses came up and I shut down really quickly." "When I took account of the current situation, I came to a clearer understanding of how I get so easily thrown off course and detached from myself."

What might be happening in the current situation that caused this reaction? Maybe we just read something, talked to someone, or saw a TV show that aroused our own sense of vulnerability. Maybe we are recovering from an illness or surgery, and we feel shaky and unprotected. Maybe—as is happening while this book is being written—there is a pandemic of epic proportions plus overt and covert forms of prejudice that might affect us if we are different from the white, heterosexual majority.

These are all good reasons to pull back from the intensity of our own feelings, to modulate by doing something else or falling back on dysregulated avoidance of the weight of all the perceived dangers. But if we continue to modulate by letting the feelings come up in small doses, a little at a time, and by creating a better TPN understanding of our own embodied processes, we just might have the courage to feel a little bit more.

This is an important function of modulated ESA. It is a transitional state that creates opportunities for allowing felt experiences to emerge in small, digestible doses. Feeling the intensity of pain of a previous loss or trauma, or feeling intense emotions like joy or anger or grief that we had spent years suppressing, is likely to overwhelm our ANS and send us back into dysregulation and even re-traumatization. One of the approaches to treating trauma, called Somatic Experiencing, refers to this process of taking small steps toward felt experience as "titration."[32]

Research done in the Department of Psychiatry at Duke University (Durham, North Carolina, USA) shows that for some people, "too much" exposure to negative emotional states all at once can cause an increase in inflammation in the body and a return to a dysregulated state. This is especially the case for those who suffer from PTSD and prior physical or emotional trauma and for people who are at risk for autonomically modulated health conditions such as cardiovascular disease, high blood pressure, and diabetes.[33] As we have seen, unresolved trauma tends to be accompanied by higher rates of physical and mental illnesses leading to low resilience (discussed in chapter 1) and a slower recovery from these trauma and illness states.

In modulated ESA, taking felt experience in these brief moments, people can build resilience step-by-step with the result that the feelings can gradually become less fearful, less likely to evoke a danger response in the amygdala, less likely to trigger inflammation and a return to dysregulated states. Practicing and repeating small doses of felt experience, perhaps with therapeutic assistance—for days, weeks, months, or years—we may begin to feel something shift.

Without conscious planning or effort, we may begin to notice a sense of being "pulled" into the difficult feelings in a way that is a little less scary on each new occasion. We are coming to that place where we are allowing our body to speak to or call to us. And this pull is likely to begin to set off longer moments of parasympathetic activation: we can feel our body begin to soften and relax instead of tightening up against the feeling.

When we open up to these feelings, we can begin to tolerate in new ways the physical pain, the terror, and maybe the memory of being frozen and helpless associated with, for example, an assault or a vehicle accident. Maybe we were unable to cry or to call out for help at that time. Maybe the perpetrator deliberately manipulated our feelings or our sexual arousal, which now brings us shame. Maybe we felt that we could have prevented the accident but were unable.

As these truly traumatic and horrible feelings begin to be permitted in awareness, we can also feel how they are connected to particular body regions where we have been holding chronic muscle tension, and how we have been avoiding activities, people, or places that may evoke the trauma memories. We might also start to feel the grief of what was taken from us and the lost years of our lives when we were cut off from parts of ourselves (like our ability to defend ourselves, to feel sexual pleasure, or to feel our aliveness). Or we might feel rage, hatred, and vengeance toward the perpetrators and facilitators who abetted our abuse.

With severe trauma it is natural that we will need a long time and some assistance to uncover all of this, even in small steps. But as this happens, the feelings and memories become gradually more tolerable. As we move closer to restorative ESA, we find that we are more able to heed the call of just being with whatever is coming up in our awareness and less willing to try to modulate or control our experience.

Eventually, there comes a moment when we are not just pulled by the feeling but sense that we are "falling into" it. There is an awareness of a big open space inside of us that has no boundary or form and is not scary. We are not dissociating—we are totally engaged in the felt experience, and all the space can be filled up with feeling. Another way of describing the sense of falling is of being called to a "state of grace." We have, at long last, made a shift from modulated into restorative ESA.

Because there is no map of the territory in between modulated and restorative ESA, there is no predicting or planning when this moment may arrive. We can create the conditions for it to happen, which usually involve being in a safe space, being in nature, or being with another living being who can connect with us unconditionally. Each person has a different way to create this safe space, and each of us has to discover what that might be in any particular moment.

For some people, this might be sitting or lying next to a loved one (a child, romantic partner, sibling, or friend) in a way that invites presence, honesty, respect, and listening. It might be having your cat or dog nestled on your lap. It might be lying in the deep grass as it sways in the wind, or sitting under the shade of a favorite tree, or being warmed by the sun on a lawn chair. It might be on a massage table receiving gentle, nondemanding touch, or talking with a trusted therapist, or having someone brush or braid our hair. It might occur in a religious service or spiritual ceremony.

For other people, it might be that the call to grace and peace comes with being in the midst of a mountain snowstorm or a windy day with waves breaking loudly over beach boulders and the sea a torrent of foam. Some of us can feel safe as we experience nature's power exploding all around us, as we sink into the comforting pull of gravity and solidity and allow the rain or snow or sea spray to wash over and cleanse us.

We may feel afraid, but the fear is restorative (see chapter 6, "Restorative ESA of Fear," p. 189) because we get that we can feel it and we can feel that we are firmly anchored to the earth and part of something bigger than ourselves. The storm is awesome, and its power allows us to confront and to be with the fear or whatever other feelings arise in the present moment. As we surrender to the storm, we surrender to the storms inside ourselves and emerge with a feeling of calm and of being healed by something much bigger than ourselves.

Moving from a modulated into a restorative state usually comes with an acceptance of all the discomfort and pain. You finally get in some profound way that the child who was left alone, or unloved, or abused, or lonely, or medically compromised, is not someone else, not just a memory that you would like to forget. That child is you!

You suffered all that, and you are still suffering for what happened to you in the past. On the one hand, there is all the grief and resentment and pain. On the other hand, there is the sense that when you stop running from your past, when you accept and allow it to be part of yourself, you no longer have to fight with yourself to hold back the feelings.

The paradox of entering genuinely restorative states of ESA is that once we reach this point of letting the demons out into the open of our felt experience without trying to control them, the result is that the difficult feelings— the pain, the grief, the shame—begin gradually to disappear. We get glimpses of this possibility at first from our thoughtful, seemingly safe perch in modulated ESA. When we can fall into restorative ESA, the fuller experience of a transcendent state is not a loss of awareness but a transformation that comes with ease and peace and letting go.

This letting go into such challenging feelings requires a sense of trust that we won't be consumed by them. So with acceptance ("these feelings are mine, they are real, they hurt, they are troubling and scary") comes a kind of surrender into this trust: that it is OK to go in there and just feel without trying to change anything.

In so doing, we are gifted with a sudden and unexpected sense of relief. We might feel like we are floating, yet we are fully present and not dissociated. There is no effort to stay present with our felt experience and no need to think about and interpret the experience because the gripping and holding on, the worry and fear, the modulated thinking, have disappeared.

This restorative ESA state is not empty. It may be filled with expansive and spacious feelings that just rise and fall like the gentle waves of a calm sea. There can be tears of joy or grief. Maybe we feel awe and transcendence. Perhaps we become aware of a deep sense of love for another person, or people as a whole. Our body and face soften. We look and feel younger.

We could, possibly for the first time in our life, come in contact with a burning rage for the hatred and crimes that people perpetrated on us, or on our ancestors, or on our neighbors (see chapter 6, "Restorative ESA of Anger," p. 184, for example). And this restorative rage just burns without any need to tense up, to retaliate, or to make things right. Restorative rage does not mean that we would not, in a modulated state, act to seek justice, restitution, or reconciliation or to set boundaries for our own safety. It means only that in this moment, we are relieved to finally get in touch with what had been hidden and scary: our own justifiable anger.

During restorative ESA, our exteroception may become heightened; we notice small things that continue our sense of peace or ease. We might notice how light comes into a room, or the color of leaves, or the voices of the people we love. These sensations fill our awareness, perhaps bringing a sense of awe or gratitude, as if the inner space we had just fallen into has expanded to include the spaces around in which everything fills our awareness and there is no need for thought or doing.

If we are in nature, we can choose to stay in the present moment. We can allow the woods, the mountains, or the sea—or even our own backyard, or the view of a tree from a window—to enter this space with us. We can feel our breathing continuing to remain relaxed and steady, our tension that wants to rise up instead fade into the background, the embrace of something bigger than ourselves enveloping and protecting us, creating a sense of oneness.

Sometimes, as we transition back into modulated ESA, as we are emerging from a state of deep rest(oration), we can catch a glimpse of liberation. We begin to sense that we might (finally!) be liberated from the judgmental eyes of other people, from our own compulsions, from our need to prove ourselves, from the fog of disconnection, or from the abyss of loneliness or depression.

Also, in this borderland as we emerge from restorative ESA into modulated ESA, we can sometimes sense that the feelings from which we are (at least momentarily) liberated are "old," that they had been lurking around inside from a childhood or adult trauma that we never had an opportunity to work through. And at the same time, we can sense that this present moment is a real and palpable part of a process of healing those old wounds.

We begin to feel restored because our tears and grief and pain over the old trauma are somehow becoming unstuck, becoming a bit less susceptible to dysregulation. We feel restored in the sense that we are coming closer to being free from the nagging physical or emotional wounds that had been in the shadows for much of our lives. And we can feel restored because a lost part of ourselves, the wounded child perhaps, can now be integrated, welcomed, and embraced as an essential component of who we are and who we are becoming.

This path toward restoration is a feeling of accepting the good and bad of our life histories. We become restored by self-compassion, by forgiving ourselves for what we could not do to protect ourselves from the trauma, and by acknowledging that we have lost a chunk of our lives because we did not have the resources, knowledge, or support about how to dive into the darkness inside.

Most likely, this restoration process will take months or years of moving between modulated and restorative ESA. We are going to need ongoing doses of self-compassion to forgive ourselves for not being able to do it all at once; for still getting dysregulated when stress and trauma states are triggered by current events; for not having any real sense of control over what happened in the past and over the unknown and unpredictable pathways of our own healing process. Our embodied selves will open and close, get dysregulated, modulated, and restored in their own time and process.

Restorative states of ESA are wonderful when they happen, but in real life these states are rare. If we lived in an environment or a culture that was more connected to the earth, to community, to a guiding sense of oneness of all things—a culture with less tech and less pressure—we might find ourselves more often in restorative states. We would not need to read a book like this one, for sure, and it would not even make sense to write such a book. We would be spending our time feeling the pulse of the earth and the vastness of the night sky.

But here we are, writing and reading, committing ourselves to the impossible duality of trying to understand intellectually restorative ESA, a state of being that is completely outside of thought and logic. In our complex culture, a written document appeals to our modulated thinking in order for us to better grasp the concrete experiences of our body. Restorative ESA is more accessible, however, when experienced and communicated in direct interpersonal connections. Modulated thinking, talking, and writing—bless their uniquely human power and potential—can lead us to the edge of restorative ESA, but we have to leave them all behind as we enter the doorway into restoration.

Summary and Conclusions

The purpose of this chapter is to help you become aware of not only the state of ESA in which you are presently living but also what it feels like to shift from one to another state of ESA. In almost all cases, we can shift from dysregulated to modulated ESA or from modulated to restorative ESA, but we cannot shift directly between dysregulated and restorative states.

This means that modulated ESA serves a crucial function as a transitional state between the other two. Modulated ESA is a "good enough" state, meaning that we can stay in this state for most of our day and continue to function reasonably well in our everyday tasks. A stable modulated state allows us to be resilient against ordinary stressors, turning them into eustress opportunities for challenge, learning new abilities, and growing our capacity to self-modulate with the normal ups and downs of living.

In spite of the importance of modulated ESA—and the remarkable gains it can bring to a person's life, perhaps after having lived for a long time in traumatic dysregulation—there is still the possibility to get even more out of living: the health-promoting and deeply fulfilling states of restorative ESA.

If you are not able right now to make this shift from modulated into restorative ESA, there are probably some really good reasons for this. In your current environment, you may not have the sense of safety that is required to let go and drop into felt experience. You may be struggling to make enough money to live. You may be living with real dangers around you like racism and other persecutions, domestic and street violence, war, refugeeism, a serious illness for you or a family member, the COVID-19 pandemic, or environmental disasters due to climate change. You may be needing all your available metabolic resources to be a caregiver, or in your job if you have one, or doing the everyday chores of cooking and cleaning and child-rearing.

Even if you can't reliably access restorative ESA right now, you can move in that direction by practicing self-forgiveness and self-compassion related to any of the conditions mentioned in the previous paragraph. This practice is enough to give your modulated ESA more frequent parasympathetic pats on the back, breaks from the routines, hugs from friends and family; have a short cry, or tell someone the honest truth without trying to make things better. You may also be able to find comfort in just knowing that when the time is right, you now have a sense of the possibility of finding restoration.

Life is all about change. Nothing stays the same for very long, including the troubles that may currently be with you. Embodied self-awareness is also about change, about shifting between states, about keeping your self-awareness sufficiently agile so you can notice where you are and make choices that lead you out of dysregulation.

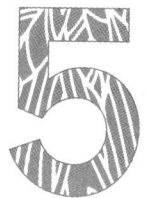

Out of the Ordinary

Pain, Eating, and Breathing during the Three States of Embodied Self-Awareness

In this chapter, we will see examples of how some of our everyday body sensations may feel in each of the three states of ESA, along with a discussion of how we shift between those states. The felt experiences reviewed in this chapter are chosen because they are common, basic, and ordinary types of body experience: pain, eating and body shape/size/appearance, and breathing.

Our awareness of these senses, and what we do with them, is also fundamental to living in a human body. Dysregulated feelings related to pain, eating, and breathing can have serious consequences for health maintenance. Becoming aware of how to shift out of dysregulated patterns and into more modulated or restorative ways to experience these senses can lead to profound changes in our well-being and our sense of ourselves in our body.[1]

Pain and Embodied Self-Awareness

Suppose that you work in front of a computer screen for many hours each day. Or perhaps you work in manufacturing and do a similar repetitive task each day that involves some strain on your eyes, or ears, muscles, or posture. You like your work, and you enjoy doing a good job and getting recognition for it. After two or five or ten years, you might discover that you are developing chronic lower back pain or carpal tunnel syndrome.

You go to the doctor, physical therapist, or chiropractor, and the analgesics, adjustments, or exercises help for a while, but the condition persists. Soon you can't concentrate on your work very well, you become grouchy with coworkers and companions, you can't do the gardening that you love, you can't lift up and hug your kids, which you love even more, and most days you don't feel like getting out of bed.

You didn't notice the wear and tear on your body because your focus was on thinking in modulated ESA: deadlines, judgments about your own performance, expectations from others that kept you thinking even after work and into the night. You imagined yourself as a valued player in a larger organization, but you could not feel your body as being sedentary and immobile most of the time.

Most people notice pain once it begins—the body's interoceptive wake-up call to pay attention to felt experience instead of to your thoughts. Hopefully, it is not too late to use relatively simple modulated ESA remedies like adjusting your posture, standing up and stretching from time to time, getting some exercise to cleanse your body of toxins, getting a massage or acupuncture or chiropractic work, or meditating to clear the mind of your compelling thoughts.

Paradoxically, even though pain is meant to be a wake-up call, it is often treated like an unwelcome guest. All we want to do is get away from it, or have that guest leave as soon as possible. Pain becomes misinterpreted by the same processes described in the previous chapters: the amygdala senses the pain as a threat, shuts down the modulatory processes of the prefrontal cortex, and shifts us into dysregulated states of self-defense—we push through the pain (fight), we avoid noticing or allowing ourselves to accept that we are in pain (flight), or we tune out all of our body sensations, pretending they don't exist (freeze/dissociation).

Embodied Self-Awareness Transforms Pain

An interview study was done on participants who suffered from chronic back pain. The researchers—from the Pain Clinic at Royal United Hospital (Bath, UK)—asked these people how they related to their own bodies. They found that the people had dissociated themselves from their embodied self-awareness. One participant reported:

> *"I never thought about my body before, I just abused it I suppose. Now I feel it and bits of it feel really weird, as if they are not part of me anymore ... the numb bits down my leg where it hurts ... they're somehow separate now."*[2]

Generally speaking, these kinds of detachment/dissociation defense strategies that attempt to suppress the feelings of pain can actually make it worse. A research study done on another group of chronic low-back-pain patients in the Department of Psychology at Rosalind Franklin University of Medicine and Science (Chicago, Illinois, USA) revealed that avoidance of emotions related to pain and to the felt experience of pain was connected to higher levels of depression and anxiety and higher ratings on pain and fatigue.[3] It is more helpful, as we saw in the previous chapter, to find ways to gradually, little by little, learn to pay attention to the pain in modulated ESA and later use the pain experience as part of the healing power of restorative ESA.

A study done at the Karolinska Institute (Stockholm, Sweden) examined changes in emotional pain during the course of a body psychotherapy treatment program for people with generalized anxiety disorder. The treatment program was designed to help clients notice where in the body they held pain and tension and to become aware of any emotions and other felt experiences that arose as they sensed the muscle tension and its related painful emotional feelings.[4]

When clients first entered the treatment program, their emotional pain was relatively dysregulated, and what they said fit the research described in the previous paragraphs: that avoiding the pain makes it worse.

"I really don't want to be sad; I used all my defenses not to feel anything and most of the time I succeeded ... and I don't like the pain, if I'm crying then I get a headache, terrible headache and I wanted to avoid that."[5]

As the body psychotherapy treatment program progressed, the first step taken by clients in moving from a dysregulated into a modulated ESA state was learning to trust themselves sufficiently to be able to let go of their dysregulated patterns of trying to avoid the painful felt experiences. Being modulated means that we can use our TPN thinking to learn and apply specific strategies that help us regulate our pain and other body symptoms. As the clients became more modulated, one of them described her experience in the following way:

"I noticed that my muscles were so tense and the impact it had on my anxiety symptoms, so now I try to counteract the tenseness in my body. I do some relaxation exercises that I learned during therapy. I have the feeling that I can control it now. Before, it was the anxiety that controlled me. Now I know directly that if I don't feel well, I get muscular pain."[6]

The shift from modulated to restorative ESA was not a main focus of this particular study, but there are some hints in the findings suggesting that at least some of the clients were, in fact, able to move beyond modulated forms of self-control and self-awareness. They were able to find more relief and let go of thinking about themselves by trusting more in their felt experiences. One participant reported,

"My self-confidence is much better today, and I don't think so much about my posture, it is more automatic. I dare to show myself in a different manner than before. I feel rather relaxed actually, everything is more unconscious. I don't have to contemplate so much."[7]

These research findings lead to a paradox. The only way out of the suffering is to jump back into it. The only way to ease the pain *and at the same time to heal the body* is to attend to and feel the pain, at first in small doses and in a modulated way. Analgesics and opiates, alcohol and psychoactive drugs, can only temporarily blunt the pain. We have to change our nervous system and the way in which our whole embodied self relates to the pain.

Another study—this one out of the Osher Center for Integrative Medicine at the University of California, San Francisco (USA)—recorded discussions during focus groups made up of eight highly skilled teachers/practitioners from different body-awareness practices (yoga, tai chi, Feldenkrais, somatic psychotherapy, Somatic Experiencing, breath therapy, and Alexander Technique). There was also another focus group containing four to six students of each of these practitioners. Participants were asked to share about how they related to their felt experiences, including the experience of pain. Many of these participants reported that—after spending months or years engaging in their particular embodied practice—they learned to be with, accept, and just feel their pain.

> *"[It was] just a huge learning for me to really pay attention to where was I getting to that edge of pain. And this—this just changed the way I started to move, in general, all the way through my day."*[8]

> *"The whole notion of sort of avoiding and pushing away unpleasant experiences that I would just do anything to, you know, avoid … Now I can just pay attention to what's happening in the moment and it's much more pleasant to get through it. And the recovery from an unpleasant experience is much quicker as well."*[9]

> *"How I feel about sensation in my body is different. It used to cause some panic in me if there was any discomfort. And now I don't immediately jump to the conclusion that I have terminal cancer if my knee hurts…. So, it's nice to have a little bit of space between the sensation and the emotional reaction to it."*[10]

The researchers concluded that for the participants in this research study,

> *a key element that changed in their relationship to their body sensations appeared to be the awareness of the differences a) between thinking about a sensation and directly sensing the sensation, and b) between a willful attention and a more relaxed, accepting and allowing attitude in their attention towards these sensations.*[11]

This is actually a very good description of making the shift from dysregulated states of pain into more modulated and perhaps even restorative states of pain awareness.

Another research study from Sweden—this one at Sahlgrenska University Hospital, Gothenburg—found that body awareness training reduced the pain and discomfort of people suffering from irritable bowel syndrome (IBS). People with IBS experience daily abdominal pain and discomfort as well as disrupted bowel function, including alternations between constipation and diarrhea. They may also have other discomforts such as headaches and painful urination. IBS often co-occurs with disorders like fibromyalgia, panic disorder, anxiety, and depression.

Participants met with a physical therapist for two hours each week for a total of twenty-four weeks. The sessions consisted of training people to move in ways that improved posture, coordination, and free breathing, with a focus on paying attention to felt sensations during the movements. Treatment with this body awareness therapy, compared to a healthy control group, showed reduction for IBS patients in gastrointestinal dysfunction and pain, reduced body tension, increased ease of movement, improved body awareness, fewer headaches, and reduced symptoms of anxiety and depression. In addition, participants reported greater self-confidence and increased coping ability, and they showed lower levels of salivary cortisol[12]—a clear shift from dysregulated into modulated ESA.

Finally I present here, for the first time, interview findings from five female clients diagnosed with low-back pain who were given sixteen sessions of Rosen Method bodywork over a period of six months. The Rosen practitioners and these five clients all lived in the East Bay region of the San Francisco Bay Area (California, USA).

In the previous chapter, I presented published findings regarding the reports of the Rosen practitioners who participated in this research, written following each session. The results of these practitioner reports showed that over the course of treatment there were no shifts between dysregulated and restorative ESA—only between dysregulated and modulated or between modulated and restorative ESA. Another result of this same research study is that clients shifted between dysregulated, modulated, and restorative ESA during each of their Rosen Method bodywork treatment sessions, with a gradual increase of restorative ESA states across sessions over time.[13]

Other published data from this study showed that the client's self-reported back pain diminished over the course of the treatments, based on daily questionnaires about their back pain, level of fatigue, and sense of well-being during the six-month treatment period. Even though their pain decreased overall, their daily reports showed big fluctuations from day to day. Some days they had high levels of pain and other days much less, showing that healing is not a linear path of improvement. There are many ups and downs along the way.[14]

Turning now to results that are reported here for the first time, during in-person interviews conducted with each client one month after completing their sixteen-session course of treatment, the clients described changes in how they related to their back pain and how that changed over time. In particular they described how, at the end of the treatment program, they were able to find a sense of restorative relief and relaxation.

> Client 1: "I notice the onset of stress-tension more, so I can choose to slow down and breathe. And, I can catch it early. I can feel it in my rib cage and I know I need to slow down. It felt like the Rosen treatments affected my nervous system on a deep level. I'm sure it helped the back pain, but it helped me unwind at a deeper level. I feel like I'm wound up a lot of the time, that I just hold things deeply in my body. And it let me relax in a way that is pretty unknown to me. I noticed that I would feel deeply relaxed and almost drift off. And when I got to that place it had a floating sensation. I likened it to snorkeling. Just suspended. I found it deeply, deeply relaxing. I just don't feel that relaxed from sleep. It nurtured me in a deeper way than I normally feel."

This client clearly speaks to the value of tuning in to her felt experience in the process of healing from back pain. She describes the beginnings of the ability to shift into finding ways to modulate her felt experiences and to notice and feel her level of stress and tension, and how that may have been related to the pain. She also describes how accepting her tension by allowing herself to feel it led eventually to recurrent access to restorative states of deep rest and relaxation.

Client 2: "My level of pain has decreased. The most beneficial thing with Rosen was it gave me a place to rest. I didn't have to do anything but lay there. This educated me about how tired I am. That has helped me to slow down or be aware of the rushing syndrome I do: awareness of pains and sensations in body and hurriedness of life and how much I don't rest. Rosen was most about rest and relaxing and heightened body awareness for me. It was a real gift in that way. The big thing I got out of it, which was unexpected, was this desire to stop rushing."

In a similar way, Client 2 made a clear connection between her dysregulated pain, tiredness, and inability to settle into herself. Like Client 1, she also discovered the health benefits of learning to modulate herself by making deliberate efforts to slow down and to stop her compulsion to rush around. And, like Client 1, she came to a place of allowing herself to enter a deeper state of relaxation and restoration.

Client 3: "Deep-seated emotional issues were causing me a lot of pain. By allowing me to just see how strangled I was around these issues and how I was holding them and the kind of damage I was doing to my body, I became willing to change my relationship to them. I stored emotions in certain areas of my body and, rather than articulate my feelings in the moment, I stored them to remain in control. It started to do damage to me. Over the years it took a toll until I was not able to function and I had to find a way to address those emotions or to experience a different way of being in the world or experience a lot of pain. That was the message I was getting from my body. We started to work more deeply when I was willing to let her [the Rosen practitioner] in. When I was willing, there was a shift."

This client, like the other two, came to the realization that she had to make a choice to open up to her felt experience and at the same to allow her practitioner to provide guidance through the challenging process of moving from dysregulation into modulation, or as she describes it, when she was willing to "let her [practitioner] in." Modulated ESA shows up as she admits to discovering how emotions were held in her body, how she learned to control their felt experience and expression, and how she had learned to remain in control.

> Client 4: "I believe that emotion attached to certain back pain, and I feel that my back pain (the lower part) is now pretty good. I didn't pay too much attention to the change, but it came on more subtly. I notice it doesn't hurt as much as before. I just feel tightness now. I always have problems with the left side, so I see it as a constant chronic pain which has gotten better. It shifted. Sometimes it's good, sometimes not so good. It depends on activities. The back pain is better because I sit less and Rosen Method released some tension. I don't feel the sharp pain anymore. Instead, I feel the muscle tightness. Those changes happened about half way through study. This work has helped me learn to open up verbally. It made me realize I need to be more vocal and speak out. I've been trying to do that more instead of keeping it all inside. And after I do it, I feel relief."

This client also noticed a link between muscle tension, pain, and holding back her emotions—the synergy that can happen in dysregulated states. She became aware of the shift between dysregulated and modulated ESA and that shift's relationship to pain reduction. Another aspect of her growing ability to be in modulated ESA is her willingness to open up and talk about her emotions. She ended the treatment period with the achievement of a relatively solid modulated ESA, with occasional flashes of some relief.

She does not feel completely "cured" and would probably need a longer period of treatment to see if it would be possible to shift more fully into restorative states of relief and relaxation. On the other hand, this person may not want to take her treatment any further. She may not feel safe enough to let go of the gains she has achieved in modulation.

As mentioned earlier, after being in pain and living in dysregulated states during a long period of suffering, the ability to modulate can feel like enough. For some people, there is no need to do any more. To take the next step into restorative ESA, we have to let go of control, which may feel like giving up our hard-earned gains. Modulated forms of control can be helpful and from a modulated state we can shift either into restorative ESA or back into dysregulated ESA.

Unless a person feels called into deeper states of safe relaxation, or until they are emotionally ready to enter the unknowable of restorative ESA, then finding regular and reliable modulation strategies can bring about a major shift in lifestyle, self-confidence, reduction of fear and stress, and diminution of trauma and pain. Accepting that modulated ESA is a big achievement and that it may be good enough for right now in one's life can bring a welcome sense of achievement and satisfaction.

Pain as an Emergent State of Embodied Self-Awareness

The research studies described in the previous section were all based on treatments that used some form of embodied self-awareness to assist clients in moving away from dysregulated states. The clients in these studies did not receive injections, manipulations, or pain meds that would have directly affected the nociceptors (pain receptors) in the body.

In ESA-based treatments, we learn how to feel, accept, and modulate the pain sensations. Pain, like all interoceptions and other felt experiences, is relatively fuzzy: hard to locate in the body and difficult to describe how it feels. The sensations from the nociceptors at the periphery of the body are not pain. Nor are the nerve impulses that travel up the spinal cord and are encoded in the brain stem, hypothalamus, thalamus, anterior cingulate cortex, and insula.

Pain is an emergent state of interoceptive "interpretation" that forms out of this complex neural network that is distributed across the whole body. *This means that pain is not a concrete thing but a state of self-awareness.*[15] Back at the nociceptors, they may be sending the same input signal to the brain, but how it is felt (intense or mild, sharp or merely achy, noticeable or not noticeable) and how we relate to it emotionally (fear or acceptance) can be changed, perhaps permanently, by becoming more aware of it in modulated or restorative ESA.

Another example of "whole-body" modulation of pain is when we laugh together with other people. As this happens, the thalamus and insula are triggered to produce neurotransmitters that have a similar chemical composition and effect on pain reduction as opioid drugs and medications.[16] Like opioid medications, these internally produced neurochemicals have the effect of increasing the threshold for the perception of pain. That means we are less likely to feel pain unless it is extremely intense. In addition to laughter, most forms of ESA practices, such as those used in the research described earlier, can trigger the production of opioid-like neurochemicals in the brain and bloodstream and thus have the same effect of altering our awareness of the experience of pain.

PAIN: SHIFTING AND HEALING

Suppose that you encounter an intense pain somewhere in your body. You notice that all you want to do is get away from that pain, to end it. You are in a dysregulated state as this is happening.

For a moment, though, you shift into a modulated state and stop trying to suppress your awareness of the pain. As you begin to feel the outlines of the pain, you notice that the muscle tension around the painful area begins to thaw, and you generate modulated thoughts to describe what is happening to yourself. The pain lessens for a bit until your nervous system can't hold on to it any longer, and again you want to escape. The dysregulated thoughts and worries come in, and the seemingly unbearable intensity of the pain and tension returns.

Then once again, you might catch yourself at the edge: the balance point between beginning to feel the pain (modulated ESA) and feeling overwhelmed by the pain (dysregulated ESA). You choose to feel the pain. This lasts for a short time, and then the shifting between modulated and dysregulated ESA begins again. With practice, you can learn to discern that on the dysregulated side the thoughts border on worries and helplessness, and on the modulated side you begin to have thoughts that you are able to hold and sense the pain and that you are getting closer to feeling it.

A moment may arrive, a kind of tipping point, when you can feel an expansion in your chest and a growing sense that you can hold more in your awareness. This is how you can tell that you are more centered in a modulated state and less likely to slip back into dysregulation. As you feel more, you might suddenly be flooded with a parasympathetic and hormonal rush, a deeper breath, and then the pain vanishes for a short period. When that happens, you know that you just made a shift from being reasonably well modulated into a brief state of restorative ESA.

It is from this "stronger" modulated state that we can then more easily open up into a restorative state. The transition from modulated to restorative ESA is radically different than the transition between dysregulated and modulated ESA. When we shift from modulated to restorative, the transition occurs suddenly and without any prior indication. One minute you are doing your best to stay focused on feeling the pain, and then, without any planning or effort, you feel yourself gradually sinking in, your breath getting slowly deeper.

And, just as suddenly, you are back in ordinary modulated reality. Your body feels normal—meaning that it has weight and tension, and the pain is there right where you left it, and the intrusive thoughts, not fully formed, are again rising like clouds with dark outlines and dark undersides, but the storm has not yet begun. There is a moment of sudden clarity in this space in between ecstasy and despair.

On each occasion that you make this transition to restorative ESA, you may be able to feel the pull into the vastness more easily; it feels safer to fall into it, and easier to soften and let go. Unlike in modulated ESA, however, you can't make a choice to stay there because there is no choosing, only being.

Dropping into restorative ESA is not like a tunnel where you know you are going somewhere and will arrive at the other end. The restorative state can't be seen or understood, so there is simply no way to think about or figure out how to get there. We only notice it when we are actually there.

Restorative ESA is a kind of medicine because the neural networks that support it are directly linked to neural, hormonal, and immune-system functions that relax, soothe, and restore. Restorative ESA medicine relies on your own body's natural resources for self-repair, and the dosage is automatically tailored to your needs.

Types of Pain Experience

Pain, as an emergent state of interoception, is not just one feeling. There are many different types of pain that have been described, although like all felt experience, it is a challenge to describe them in narrative thought or language. Justin Schmidt, an entomologist at the University of Arizona in Tucson, studies stinging insects. Unlike other entomologists, Schmidt has indulged in felt experience by allowing himself to be stung by many different types of critters. In his book *The Sting of the Wild: The Story of the Man Who Got Stung for Science* and other writings, he has developed an evocative language for these experiences.

> *Club-horned wasp, Pain Level 0.5, "Disappointing. A paper clip falls on your bare foot."*
>
> *Anthophorid bee, Pain Level 1, "Almost pleasant, a lover just bit your earlobe a little too hard."*
>
> *Termite-raiding ant, Pain Level 2, "The debilitating pain of a migraine contained in the tip of your finger."*
>
> *Maricopa harvester ant, Pain Level 3, "After eight unrelenting hours of drilling into that ingrown toenail, you find the drill wedged into the toe."*[17]

Of course, each person will experience the same insect bite in a different way because pain is not an objective, real "thing" but rather a state of awareness. A notable consequence of pain being a state of awareness is that emotional pain and physical pain activate the exact same areas of the insula and the anterior cingulate cortex. These same interoceptive pain regions that activate when stung by an insect also become activated when people experience social rejection or a breakup with a romantic partner.[18]

We could say that emotional pain is just another type of pain experience, but pain, like all interoceptive feelings, is almost always both a physical and an emotional experience. If we trip over something and hurt our foot, in addition to feeling physical pain we are likely to also be angry or disappointed with ourselves or with someone else who is convenient to blame. ("Why did you leave that box in the hallway where I couldn't see it until I hurt myself? Now look what you've done!!" "I'm so stupid: I was talking on my phone and wasn't paying attention to where I was walking.")

Conversely—and here is what most people don't fully appreciate—emotional pain doesn't just hurt psychologically; it hurts somewhere in our body. With a physical pain, there is an obvious link between the psychological experience of pain and a physical location in the body. This is because the information from the nociceptors where we got injured is sorted by the thalamus into distinct body locations. The marvel of the nervous system is that even though interoception is largely an inferential creation of whole-body neural complexity, we feel in 3D: the pain is "in" the knee or wherever.

If there really is an economy of pain networks that includes both physical and emotional pain, and if physical pain has a body location, then this simple syllogism leads to the conclusion that emotional pain must have a physical location in the body. In what way might emotions be embodied?

All emotions have a component of muscle movements, our emotional expressions. Even if we try to hide our feelings, there will be micro-momentary muscular activation. The anterior cingulate is located right next to the premotor area, which begins the process of forming an emotional expression in the body. The premotor area connects to the motor cortex above it and then—via the brain stem and spinal cord—back to the specific muscles of expression.

In this case, emotional pain may be located in those places in the body where an expression was meant to happen but failed to materialize because we suppressed it. We might feel like screaming at the person who left that object in the hall, the object that we tripped over, but we didn't actually scream, and in fact, we didn't take our anger out on the person. So we might have residual muscle pain in the neck, throat, and jaw (from holding back the angry scream).

That neglectful person, then, is experienced as a pain in the neck or a pain in the butt (the suppressed urge to kick?) or as being fed up (a feeling in the chest and gut that we are going to burst?). Deeper insults go deeper into the body. Rage and hatred are the ultimate gut feelings, down in the bowels (I'm so mad I could puke; you make me sick to my stomach).

The studies cited at the beginning of this section were about social rejection. Where is that felt in the body? A broken heart? Downhearted? Is love and its loss more than metaphorically connected to the heart and chest? Yes, says a large body of research from behavioral medicine and health psychology.[19] Similarly, the emotion of disgust often shows up as feelings of nausea, wanting to vomit, and digestive upset and irritation.[20]

The sense of safety that comes from being in the company of loved ones is created partly by vagal-parasympathetic activation, which promotes an easy and relaxed integration of breathing and heart rate, both of which are located in the chest. Feelings of insecurity get the heart and the breath out of sync, activate the sympathetic nervous system as if we were dealing with a threat (elevated heart rate and blood pressure), and can create a sense of unease in the chest, and even pain.

People who have been traumatically hurt by others—especially in childhood—often have retracted chests and downcast postures that are muscular ways of protecting the heart and closing off the self from fully engaging with others for fear of being hurt again. And people in insecure relationships are more likely to have cardiovascular (and other health) problems than those who are more secure.

With physical pain, we'd be in big trouble if we could not locate it in our body via the direct inner experience of feeling it. How would we (our brain) know how to deal with the pain (how to move, how to sit, or how to lie down without further injury) in the absence of a location and a direct interoception?

In order to get over grief, resolve anger, and even embrace happiness, we have to feel those things in the body. We are quick to access the body locations of pleasurable feelings (food, drink, sex, warmth, touch), so why not also let ourselves go to the places of emotional pain? Yes, it hurts for a while, but then—miraculously—there can be restorative relief and the emergence of a new perspective on ourselves and others.

Unwanted pain also arises from memories of painful or traumatic experiences. The same process applies to remembered pain as to emotional and physical pain in the present moment. The more we are able to feel safe enough to allow ourselves to reexperience traumatic memories, the easier they become to tolerate.[21]

Many types of trauma therapy provide the opportunity to reexperience such memories, at first in small modulated doses to give the felt-experience neural networks the opportunity to stay present with the experience even for a brief period of time in modulated ESA. Gradually, as our body begins to accept that the trauma is part of our past experience, we have the opportunity to stay with the memories for longer periods, just as in the experiential exercise in the previous sidebar.

This likely creates the same kinds of endogenous opioids in the insula that, along with the guidance of a trusted friend or therapist, allow us to fully reexperience the memory in a way that brings restoration and healing. At some point in this process, the fear of the painful memory lessens, and the memory itself begins to fade into an adaptive and healthy form of forgetting. We are less troubled by what happened to us in the past, and we have more confidence that we are able to feel and tolerate other kinds of painful memories.[22]

Eating, Body Image, and Embodied Self-Awareness

How we eat and how we feel about our body size and shape can be understood, like pain, from the perspective of the three states of embodied self-awareness. Food involves both thinking and felt experience, beginning with the acts of acquiring and preparing the groceries or getting food from a restaurant, and continuing with the act of eating and the resulting experience of the journey of that food through the mouth, the digestive tract, and exiting our body through urinary and fecal elimination.

Food is also intimately bound up with our sense of self. What and how we eat becomes part of our identity (fast-food junkie, a foodie who likes to try different kinds of food, a follower of a particular diet like keto or paleo, a specialist in one or more kinds of ethnic foods, a health-food aficionado). And these factors are intimately bound up with our body image, cultural norms, how other people see us, and the way we feel about the others' gaze.

This section is not about nutrition, diet, or the connection between food and health. There are many other resources on these topics. Rather, this section is about our embodied awareness of ourselves in relation to food and eating, and about how we can cultivate our ability to notice our states of ESA and facilitate shifting from potentially dysregulated patterns of eating into more modulated or even restorative eating.

Dysregulated Eating

The growing use of computers, televisions, tablets, smartphones, and video games means that recreation has turned increasingly indoors, become sedentary, and has the effect of numbing the body and its sensations as we are engaged in these activities. Many people consume food in the same way that they consume devices: without paying much attention to felt experience. This pattern of eating eventually shows up in the form of a variety of eating disorders.

By all measures, eating disorders are epidemic in industrialized nations. This has been especially hard on youth, with a dramatic worldwide rise in adolescent eating disorders. The growing middle class in most nations has brought with it conditions that create opportunities for the overuse and misuse of food.

On the one hand, there is year-round worldwide availability of a huge diversity of food, including highly processed foods. On the other hand, there is increased pressure on families to work more to maintain their middle-class standard of living. That leads to less free time to enjoy meals together or to have the opportunity for family food preparation and social sharing. The situation is worse for people living with lower income levels and poverty. There is an increasing reliance on fast and processed foods containing high levels of salts, sugars, fats, and carbohydrates, which are cheap, give a feeling of fullness, and subdue hunger at least for several hours.

In the most common forms of eating disorders, food is a way to suppress felt experiences including unwanted emotions such as frustration, discouragement, muscle tension, fatigue, pain, hunger and thirst, and worries about income loss, food supply, clothing, and body image. There are two basic dysregulated eating strategies to suppress felt experience: either to eat too much or eat too little.

In the case of those who eat too little (presuming they are not facing food shortages or starvation), they are focused on external images of the ideal body or behaving in accordance with peer-group expectations. They are preoccupied with being negatively evaluated because of the way they look, and the stress of how they appear to others suppresses their own felt experiences about what is good and healthy for themselves.

Eating too little can become chronic in the case of anorexia nervosa (self-starvation). Anorexic teens show a typical profile of higher levels of sympathetic nervous system arousal, which suppresses emotions and the interoceptive experiences involved with eating.[23]

Those who eat too much focus on the food itself. If food is present, no matter what type of food, they are likely to indulge in eating it. These individuals suppress the interoceptive awareness required for healthy modulation of food intake, such as by not being able to feel fullness or satiety, ignoring the gastrointestinal distress and indigestion that often accompany overeating, or taking a regular dosing of antacids or other digestive aids.[24]

In a wide range of populations and in many different research studies, binge eating has been linked to life stress coupled with suppression of body sensations and emotions and with negative mood.[25] For people with binge-eating disorders, foods high in sugars and calories activate their insula while healthier foods do not. This means that these unhealthy foods are the only ones that can create a felt experience of satisfaction. In people who eat healthy diets, on the other hand, the insula is more attuned to a wider range of felt experiences related to taste, smell, texture, and nourishment in foods.

For people who have healthy eating habits, there is a functional connection between the insula and the orbitofrontal cortex that regulates feelings of attraction or repulsion toward food. This circuit is linked to the anterior cingulate cortex, which regulates motivation toward healthy tasting and smelling food and away from foods high in animal fats, added sugars, and other carbohydrates. This functional connectivity between the insula and prefrontal cortex creates the possibility for modulated and restorative ESA during food preparation and intake.

This familiar neural network for felt experience becomes dysregulated in people with eating disorders.[26] Their dysregulated neural networks somehow fail to detect that some types of dietary choices—fresh fruits and vegetables, lean meats, "good fats" like olive oil and avocado, and foods low in sugar and salt—are actually food sources.

Of course, people who eat too much can categorize in their TPN that healthy foods are things that can be eaten by humans. But these are not foods that people with this kind of eating disorder would willingly choose because they simply do not "show up" in felt experience as tasty or fulfilling.

It gets worse. Either filling up with too much food or entering a state of semi-starvation creates changes in the nervous system that lead to feeling soporific, depressive, or anxious. Clinical case reports reveal that these states further suppress felt experience that could lead to healthier food choice. The excess food or starvation "high" becomes a dysregulated ESA state in which the food is used as an addictive palliative.[27]

In youths, binge eating sometimes co-occurs with other forms of dysregulated ESA such as self-injurious behavior (e.g., burning and cutting) because these strategies provide at least temporary relief from negative emotions and ruminations.[28] In some but not all cases, teens who resort to these methods of self-soothing in the face of dysregulated feelings may have suffered from childhood trauma, including but not limited to physical abuse, loss of parental support, shaming about body image, and sexual abuse.[29]

Women and girls, on average, suffer more from eating disorders and are more likely to feel like they have to make an effort to fit in to social pressures. Research done at the Division of Adolescent and Young Adult Medicine, University of California, San Francisco (USA), shows that only 22 percent of young males, compared to 80 percent of young females, develop some form of eating disorder related to appearance. These eating-disordered boys and men rank high on gender stereotypes and worry about their muscularity. They overeat, abuse alcohol, and spend excessive amounts of time indulging in risky forms of exercise—such as heavy weight lifting, rollerblading, and skateboarding—to bulk up to increase their size and strength and enhance their appearance.[30]

Research done at Bard College (Annandale-on-Hudson, New York, USA) reveals that almost all young women overestimate their body size, feel too fat even if they are normal weight, and are or have been on some kind of diet; most of these women will gain back the weight once they stop the diet because dieting can predispose them to binge eating.[31]

Most girls and women feel a pressure to look good in order to please others. Researchers at the University of Sussex (UK) showed that girls as young as five years old were more likely to endorse statements showing dissatisfaction with their own body after experimental exposure to thin Barbie dolls and to thin female images in the media.[32] As girls reach adolescence, body dissatisfaction can be exacerbated or lessened, depending upon whether their peer group and family are focused on external ideals and criticism or an embodied awareness-based sense of personal well-being.[33]

For example, women prone to overeating, compared to those who were not, were more likely to order dessert at a restaurant following a filling meal if other people in the group were planning to order dessert.[34] Dysregulated eating patterns such as binge eating and anorexia can also be adopted because of wanting to fit in and model the behavior of other girls in a peer group. The effort to please others outweighs the signals from one's own body, suppressing felt experience.[35]

You might think that the effort to look good would have salutary effects on a person's relationship to food. To look good, the optimal strategy would be to eat a balanced diet that is healthy and nourishing: a food program that feels good in a modulated or restorative way in the shopping, preparing, and eating process. The reality for many women and for some men is that their attention is directed outward to what others think about their body and away from what their body feels like and what their body needs to be healthy.

Negative body image has a direct impact on self-esteem. Studies done at Pennsylvania State University (University Park, USA) show that women who feel less satisfied with their breast size, their facial attractiveness, and their sex appeal are less likely to express their opinion (on any topic) in public. They are less confident in their ability to succeed, and they feel more self-conscious and more ashamed of their bodies. They are also less likely to feel satisfied in their sexual relationships and show less assertiveness regarding their own sexual needs.[36]

Women who are more susceptible to eating disorders are more likely to engage frequently in behaviors collectively referred to as "body checking." These behaviors include frequent self-inspection of the whole body shape and size in front of a mirror; pinching the flesh of the stomach or arms to check for bulges, sags, and fatness; and checking the fit of rings on the fingers.[37] Compared to most men who go to gyms to bulk up, when women exercise in environments with mirrors, they actually feel less positive about themselves, offsetting any mood and health-improvement benefits of exercise.[38]

Again, we come to the paradoxical conclusion that the very worries about appearance that should contribute to healthy eating and exercising actually suppress felt experience and contribute to the development of an appearance that creates even more dissatisfaction and a lower sense of self-worth. And again, one of the main effective pathways out of this particular vicious circle of dysregulated ESA is to cultivate experiences of more modulated and restorative patterns of eating in which improving how we feel takes precedence over social norms and physiological attractions to dysregulated eating. Shifting into more modulated eating patterns requires learning to pay attention and to enjoy food sensations that are connected to healthier diets.

Modulated and Restorative Eating

For optimal health and rejuvenation, we all need modulated ESA practices such as exercise, rest, healthy foods, some time to feel deeply into ourselves, and meaningful and emotionally expressive human interpersonal contact. Under stress, however, these modulated techniques can be easily ignored. Maybe we can tell ourselves that we don't want to exercise or that we don't want to be around other people. We do, however, have to eat. It's required. So how can we make the process of eating fit into the scope of a modulated

ESA practice, one that is both self-sustaining and adds to our ability to be healthy and productive?

Since eating disorders are associated with emotional suppression, clinical work with people who suffer with eating disorders usually relies on the gradual development of shifting into more modulated forms of emotion regulation. This might include emotional intelligence strategies that use thought patterns to identify negative emotions and self-evaluations and to create strategies for understanding how negative emotion may lead to dysregulated eating and self-injury. Further cognitive strategies that boost self-understanding and self-compassion can be developed to help people reduce their temptation to eat as a means for self-calming.[39] These strategies are based in cultivating forms of TPN thought that help in tracking emotions and logically understanding the link between emotion and food choices.

Another approach to a more healthy pattern of eating, based in felt experience rather than TPN thinking, is called *intuitive eating*. This has three dimensions: (1) developing a reliance on internal hunger and satiety cues; (2) eating for sensory pleasure and health-sustaining reasons rather than to suppress negative emotions; and (3) unconditional permission to eat when hungry, with no self-denial. People who score higher on tests of intuitive eating are more attuned to the interoceptive signals of healthy and pleasurable eating.[40]

Similarly, young children who enjoy food more and are less picky about food choices have parents who emphasize enjoyment of food preparation and the process of making and eating good foods. Picky eating is also reduced when parents allow children to make their own food choices, both in preparing and eating—that is, when there is less pressure from parents about what and how to eat, less judgment about looks, and more of an emphasis on what feels good to the child.[41]

Modulated and restorative ESA in relation to eating can start at the market. How do you go about buying food? Are you looking for something prepared, easy, quick, and cheap? Do you pay attention to sugars, salts, calories, and fats in the ingredients? Is your shopping for food in-and-out, just another errand in a busy day? As you are shopping, are you thinking about the preparation process, about who is going to be sharing your meal, or about your other errands and tasks?

If you take a few extra minutes and put the thoughts in the background of awareness, you can have a wonderfully sensual experience in the market and later at home when you prepare the food. Fresh fruits and vegetables come in great varieties of colors, tastes, textures, and smells. Can you let your choices be guided by all your senses, not just your economic sense of value or your conceptual thoughts about what seems easiest or best for pleasing other people?[42]

Buying and preparing food using all your felt experiences can be restorative: the zen of shopping and chopping. Maybe you don't have time to meditate or exercise or get a massage, but you can use the necessity of eating to pull you back into your body and its senses. This sensory and sensual connection to and through food can be expanded if you share foraging, cooking, and eating with friends and family.

Food brings people together like nothing else, especially if your life is otherwise spent away from these cherished people. Researchers at the University of Illinois (Urbana-Champaign, USA) and Yale University (New Haven, Connecticut, USA) suggest that having regular family meals increases child health and promotes social and cognitive development, in part because of the shared activity that accompanies eating slowly and with others.[43]

Another form of restorative eating is the Slow Food movement.[44] This approach provides techniques for relating to food at all levels: from seeds to harvesting to sustainability to preparation and consumption. The Slow Food movement aims to utilize food in a way that will nourish your senses with pleasure and purpose, sending cascades of those opioid-like mood-elevating neurotransmitters and hormones through your system.

Slow Food means to shop and eat while paying attention to your felt experience, and we know that restorative felt experience requires us to slow down in order to really feel. Instead of food shopping and preparation being done as a modulated chore, you can find ways in which food will actually recharge your batteries and restore your mood, health, and interpersonal connections.

CHOCOLATE DECADENCE

Chocolate Decadence is the name of a particularly rich and creamy flourless chocolate torte made usually with butter, eggs, maybe some cream and almond meal, and of course dark and velvety melted chocolate with a high percentage of cacao and low amount of sugar. Dark chocolate also contains high levels of healthful anti-oxidants. If you don't like chocolate or cakes, then substitute some form of food indulgence that is reasonably healthy and has the possibility of making you feel good.

Modulated ESA: You are eating your slice of Chocolate Decadence while talking to someone, or reading, or checking email, or none of these things but you've got a lot on your mind. In your mouth, chewing, it's definitely chocolaty and creamy, it's familiar, it settles into a mental list of formerly consumed dessert treats and merits an imagined spreadsheet of comparison and categorization. You might be planning how you eat: not too fast, and you have to discern how long to wait between bites as you are moving toward the completion of eating this (wow!) increasingly tiny slice.

Maybe you are telling yourself that you are really enjoying this and tasting it. You are convincing yourself in modulated TPN or DMN thought that you are not rushing, and perhaps thinking things like "It's really good," or "Wonderful," or "I need to thank X for making this awesome dessert." You might also be thinking about when and how to take a picture of the slice (pre-eaten, one bite taken out maybe?) to post on social media and what you plan to say about it.

Each bite lasts only seconds, then you count and wait, take another bite the same as the last, moving another step toward finishing. Now it's gone and you continue the thoughts, telling yourself that you are full and complete, or that you want more, or that you have to get up and do the dishes or pay the bill, and move on to the next thing. Maybe you do want another slice?

Restorative ESA: Fattiness spreads over the surface of your tongue as it warms in your mouth and melts, a feeling of blessing, hope, soothing in how it envelops and softens the tongue into a sense of receptivity, like the tongue can just rest peacefully and contentedly in the bottom of your mouth. And then the chocolate flavors hit their notes along the tongue and register as cinnamon, cloves, earth, cacao, coffee, bitter, and sweet.

These flavors land right in the pleasure centers of your nervous system and spread into a relaxation response with a deep sigh and an aphrodisiacal tinge of hormones of full-body warmth. Then come the grace notes against the swelling fatty base; a chocolate rush on the tongue and then the whole mouth and maybe you haven't even felt the urge to chew but only to move your tongue in and out like a baby's sucking motions that express the flavors and textures of the (clearly now) decadent morsel.

And then the fading, the waning, the loss felt on swallowing, the ending that slowly and inexorably emerges and blossoms as the fat dissolves into tasteless saliva with, yes, a few lingering essences still adhering to the grooves of the tongue and between the teeth and evoking a memory of what had been, just moments ago, filling your entire body.

And in this way, your present-moment, nonthinking felt experience "decides" when to take another bite, when to feel, when to swallow, each bite a timeless lifetime, a shameless ecstasy: really totally without shame and full of a contagious feeling of mischievousness and forbidden pleasure. Hmmm. Yes, a shameless ecstasy of softness, of sparks of flavor, each completely in itself and completely true, and strangely there is no desire, no waiting for something else to happen, no anticipation; only your own melting and softening as if you were in the arms of a completely safe and trusted loved one.

It actually turns out that consumption of dark chocolate—but not other forms of chocolate—in moderate amounts decreases symptoms of depression, according to a study conducted by a multinational consortium of researchers (UK, Australia, Canada, Turkey, Austria, Spain, China, Italy, and USA) done on 13,626 men and women over the age of twenty. Chocolate can produce a response that is similar to the euphoria from cannabis. It also contains phenylethylamine, a neuromodulator related to mood regulation and depression. Dark chocolate, in particular, contains higher levels of flavonoids that have been shown to reduce inflammation and decrease depression.[45]

You may have noticed that one of the distinctions between modulated and restorative ESA in the Chocolate Decadence example is allowing ourselves to experience the absence of taste and flavor between bites of cake, and to be open to this part of the eating experience just as much as when our mouth is suffused with almost erotic flavors. Mark Epstein, in his book *Thoughts without a Thinker*, writes:

> *When I am in the middle of a particularly delicious mouthful of food, I can see my desire to move another helping into my mouth as the flavor fades, before I have finished chewing and swallowing … When I permit myself to taste the faded remnants of a mouthful of food, I am surrendering my need for continual pleasure and opening to an authentic appreciation of my actual situation.*[46]

Another approach to working with eating disorders that, like intuitive eating, is based in the felt experience part of ESA, is to focus interventions not on dieting or eating per se but more generally on cultivating an ability to settle into felt experience. A study from Deakin University and several hospital outpatient eating disorder treatment clinics in Melbourne, Australia, for example, analyzed the personal journal writings of twenty eating-disordered women who were enrolled in a twelve-week yoga program.[47]

The women in this study received weekly sessions of hatha yoga, which is not an aerobic exercise. The program had the goals of encouraging these participants to create for themselves a daily yoga routine. The foci of the yoga classes were: (1) interoceptive and proprioceptive body awareness by feeling the differences between movement and stillness (*asana*); (2) awareness of breathing patterns (*pranayama*); and (3) mindful eating meditation.

For each meal, participants were asked to remove all distractions (such as TV, books, smartphones), to pay attention to the amount of food placed in the mouth and how it tastes, and to wait until swallowing that mouthful before taking more food (like the restorative-ESA way of eating Chocolate Decadence).

In the early phases of the yoga study, one of the participants reported the kind of disconnection from her own body awareness that was discussed in the previous section on dysregulated eating. She said, "How is it possible to be so unconscious of the way you appear, yet be so obsessed with it? I think I disassociate from my body 90% of the time." Another said, "I hate what I'm doing to myself. I recognize it as self-punishment/mutilation but my intellect and emotions aren't communicating with each other. Body feels awful. Aches + pains all over, bloated, constipated, flatulent, headaches, nausea, puffy ankles."[48]

By the end of the treatment program, the women reported a more healthy connection to food and to feelings of self-empowerment about food choices. They became more aware of themselves in the present moment, such as by reducing the quantity of food eaten in one meal and decreasing their speed of eating. Their body image improved and they felt more self-confident.

From the perspective of this book, the most salient aspect of this yoga program was that the leaders made a deliberate effort not to offer dietary advice and not to discuss in any way the issue of weight loss. No special diet? No harping about weight loss? Instead, this yoga program was all about cultivating restorative ESA, our ability to stay connected to our interoceptive sensations and emotional states without intervening thoughts or judgments.

With respect to food, this means slowing down to feel how it smells, looks, and tastes. Restorative ESA means being in the present moment with the feeling of food moving down the esophagus and feelings of hunger and satiety, empty or full. No matter what is on your plate or who is around you, restorative ESA is the cultivation of an inner felt sense of when to eat, how to enjoy it, and when to stop eating.

Similar to the yoga intervention, a study done at Indiana State University (Terre Haute, USA) examined something called the Mindfulness-Based Eating Awareness Training program. This program, like the yoga program, also gave participants more self-confidence in making healthy food choices that were related to the cultivation of an inner "wisdom" and trust in the body. This included teaching the ability "to look inside oneself for how to make choices about what to eat, when to eat, how much to eat, rather than depending on the strict rules of the dieting mentality."

Learning to use this wisdom also involved "letting go of self-judgment and searching in a flexible way to develop new patterns of eating and food choice." Not only did the participants begin to make healthier food choices similar to those in the yoga study, but they also spontaneously reported more restorative experiences. These included enjoying life more and taking time to feel "the wind in my hair or sun on my face."[49]

Taking the lessons of these programs, as well as what we know about modulated and restorative ESA, how could we use our felt experience to know when it is time to stop eating? Feeling full is one way, but this is not always easy to sense, especially when there is more food available or if others around you are still eating. Another way is to notice when eating begins to feel effortful. At some point in the meal, the pleasures of taste, smell, and color of the food begin to diminish. We might become aware of the effort of lifting the food to our mouth, or the effort of chewing and swallowing. It is highly likely that if you stop eating when you sense this effort, you will actually notice the feeling of fullness that you did not notice at first.

Another felt-sense pathway to avoid overeating is by getting more comfortable with the feeling of hunger. By the end of the twelve-week yoga program described earlier, for example, some participants reported that they actually enjoyed a newfound feeling of hunger. "I feel peaceful and hopeful. I'm eating like a normal person, enjoying what I eat and not obsessing like usual. I am not currently afraid of feeling hungry. Sometimes I enjoy the feeling of hunger as my body digests the lovely healthy food I've just fed it."[50]

The only problem with intuitive eating, yoga, and mindful eating interventions is that not everyone may be likely to want to engage in this and other forms of group activity if they are sensitive to others' body-image concerns about them. Under these conditions, a more concrete approach that uses TPN processes by giving prescriptive practices is likely to work better in order to begin to build a modulated approach to eating. This might include keeping a food journal (along with notes about the felt experience of shopping, preparing, and eating) or maintaining a regular meal pattern with fewer junk-food snacks in between. These modulated TPN strategies are important transitional steps as people begin to learn to feel safe enough to access and trust their own felt experience.[51]

Whatever a person does to change their habits of eating and find a way to be comfortable in their own body will only work if their chosen practice becomes a part of their regular, daily routine. Practice yoga. Practice meditation. Practice tai chi. Practice moving with awareness. Practice exercising with awareness. Practice eating with awareness of the felt experience. Practice meal planning, journaling, or whatever works for you. The key is developing a new habit of staying in touch with ourselves so that we can modulate our thought process, weight, and body-image strategies so as to move toward a greater sense of confidence in our own choices and in how we look and feel.

Practice anything that helps you stay aware and keeps you coming back after you (inevitably but hopefully only temporarily) lose yourself. The more often you practice, the more you help your body create and strengthen spinal and brain neural transmission speeds and connections all along the pathways for felt experience. This means that each time you come back to the next practice session, you will be able to access any type of embodied feeling more quickly (including all the feelings around eating) and be able to stay in the present moment for a longer period, with the possibility of eventually arriving in a state of restorative ESA.[52]

Breathing and Embodied Self-Awareness

Take ten or fifteen minutes and notice your breathing as you go about your normal life. You'll probably discover that there are times when you are involuntarily holding your breath. Try to figure out why you might be doing this. Usually, breath holding occurs under stress or threat. It can also occur when we are anticipating something or wanting something to happen: this is the origin of the phrase "Don't hold your breath!" when expected things may not come true.

Holding your breath doesn't mean a complete cessation of breathing, although that sometimes occurs during nail-biting moments in real life and while immersed in the virtual world of games, fiction, and film. More typically, holding your breath means that your breathing is restricted because of increased tension in the muscles responsible for breathing. These include the thoracic diaphragm—a large flat muscle that stretches across the lower ribs and sits just under the heart and on top of the stomach—and some of the abdominal, chest, neck, and shoulder muscles.

The topic of breathing is introduced in this chapter because, of all the body systems, the breath is the most reliable indicator of our state of ESA. Breathing changes as we shift between dysregulated, modulated, and restorative ESA. Unlike pain and feelings about our body image, which change relatively slowly and with a lot of practice, breathing changes can happen very quickly. So, learning to notice our breath is one of the simplest means of assessing our state of ESA.

The primary muscle movements related to inhalation are the stretching of the dorsal intercostal muscles and the downward expansion of the diaphragm. The intercostals are tiny muscles between each rib bone that increase or decrease the spaces between the ribs. The dorsal intercostals are located in the back of the rib cage. You might have to take a moment to notice that your diaphragm expands downward into your belly when you breathe in. This gives the lungs, which do not have any muscle tissue in them, more space to expand in the chest as the air comes in. The diaphragm is always the first muscle to contract, followed by the intercostals, and later by accessory breathing muscles in the neck and upper chest that lift and open the upper part of the rib cage to allow the lungs to expand upward.

During relaxed restorative breathing, these muscles are moving primarily when we inhale, expanding the chest cavity to allow the lungs to take in air. These movements occur without effort or thought. Relaxed restorative exhalation, on the other hand, is primarily passive. The principal muscles of inhalation simply relax and return to a resting state, allowing the chest to contract and the carbon dioxide (CO_2) from the blood-gas exchange to flow out of the body. Relaxed breathing also has a detectable "expiratory pause," a complete cessation of movement and a total relaxation in the breathing muscles at the end of an exhalation. At this point in the respiratory cycle, just before the next in-breath, all the breathing muscles are totally at rest and without residual tension.

A longer expiratory pause indicates greater relaxation in a more restorative state of ESA, while a short or nonexistent expiratory pause indicates effortful breathing usually associated with modulated or dysregulated ESA. As you spend a while noticing your breathing patterns, you can pay particular attention to this special moment between the end of the exhale and beginning of the next inhale.

Relaxed breathing accompanies states of restorative ESA, while effortful breathing occurs in states of sympathetic activation during modulated or dysregulated ESA. In these two states, there is *contraction of the breathing muscles through both the inhalation and the exhalation*, and generally higher levels of muscle tension throughout the body. Exhalation in these sympathetic states is not a letting go of effort but a continuation of muscular activation that usually goes with a reduced expiratory pause. With effortful breathing, we might have a feeling of having to force the air out of the body or not being able to get enough air into the body.

Holding our breath is most likely to occur at the end of an inhalation. An example would be when we take a big breath before swimming with our head underwater. When we come out of the water, there is no relaxed pause at the end of the expiration because we are hungry for air.

Under conditions of mental stress—such as when we're engaged in a demanding phase of thinking and problem solving using our modulated TPN—our breathing typically shows a different pattern. Our inhalation and exhalation are more forced, our respiration rate is higher than normal, the amount of air inhaled and exhaled on each breath is lower than normal, and the amount of expelled CO_2 is reduced, leaving the body in a slightly more toxic state and without a rest period at the end of the exhalation.

Higher stress levels, such as during fearful and anxious moments of dysregulation or an episode of pain, can lead to even more extreme increases in respiration rate and thus hyperventilation without a complete clearing of CO_2.[53] The felt experience of lower blood oxygen and higher blood CO_2, coupled with a felt lack of control over an increasing respiration rate, can feed back into the autonomic nervous system (ANS) stress-response system, creating panic attacks and other physiological symptoms such as dysregulated anxiety and increased heart rate (see chapter 6, "Fear/Anxiety," p. 186).[54]

Dysregulated states can be precipitated in our breathing when we are around people who are smoking or there is environmental smoke, dust, allergens like pollen, or pollution in the air. In these cases of inhaling toxins, the constriction in breathing begins in the interoceptors located in the nostrils. These receptors trigger a whole-body neural network that creates an involuntary partial closing of the nasal passages. This restricts air flow by narrowing the passageway for air coming into the lungs, setting off a cascade of peripheral receptors in the nose and throat that detect CO_2 and lead to feelings of stress and what is called *air hunger*.

Air hunger results in feelings of fear, anxiety, and panic and can predispose us to hyperventilation, an increase in breathing frequency. Hyperventilation changes the neuro- and blood chemistry of the body and can result in muscle spasms and chest, heart, and gastrointestinal pain and distress. Extreme hyperventilation is a health risk that often requires medical intervention to restabilize breathing.[55]

Medically, air hunger occurs in people who experience acute respiratory distress syndrome such as those affected by asthma, emphysema, viral lung infections such as COVID-19, and in ICU settings where people are intubated following surgeries or put on a respirator to regulate breathing. In these cases, not only are there short-term feelings of panic but there is a high probability of longer-term post-traumatic stress and anxiety disorders that result from respiratory illnesses and respiratory-related medical procedures.[56]

The breathing patterns described so far are all involuntary physiological responses to our sense of safety, stress, or trauma. But breathing can be both involuntary and voluntary. We can hold our breath intentionally. We can take deeper breaths. We can use our modulated TPN thinking to remind ourselves to breathe when we are stressed or scared.

Psychophysiological research has shown that breath awareness and conscious efforts to control breathing patterns can activate the parasympathetic nervous system and allow for a shift from dysregulated ESA (as in pain, anxiety, addictions, depression, and trauma) to a more productive and purposeful modulated ESA.[57] Breath control has long been used to reduce pain in childbirth and reduce the need for medical intervention.[58] Yoga, tai chi, meditation, and other disciplines teach conscious breath observation and control as a way to reduce stress.

And we can voluntarily notice and slow our breathing in challenging situations. In the interview study cited earlier in this chapter done at the Osher Center for Integrative Medicine at the University of California, San Francisco (USA), one of the interviewees specifically mentioned using breath control as a way to relieve dysregulated states:

> *"When I'm in a stressful situation ... when the stress arises, you know, when you get to the airport and your plane is delayed nine hours and there's no flights and no hotels and everyone else is sort of screaming, I don't join in that. Now I can just see 'oh I'm feeling a little agitated, time to start breathing.'"*[59]

When we use conscious awareness of breathing and efforts to control and modulate our breathing, we are shifting ourselves out of dysregulated and into a more modulated state of ESA. But you don't need to specifically train your breathing to change your breathing patterns from dysregulated to modulated.

Just becoming aware of any felt experience and allowing yourself to be with it for at least a short period of time before you start to think about it will lead to more relaxed breathing. In the airport example from the previous quote, this would mean to modulate ourselves by making a deliberate effort to sit, slow down, maybe close our eyes, stop thinking, and just feel the rising sense of panic or anxiety. As we do that, our breathing will just naturally return to a more relaxed, parasympathetic pattern.

As we've seen in many other examples in this book, during modulated ESA when we take a few moments to simply feel ourselves, we are rewarded with a brief visit to a parasympathetic state. Parasympathetic states induce the felt sense of calming down, which derives from a relaxation of the muscles that are controlled by the ANS (see Figure 2.4, p. 63), including the diaphragm and gut muscles that may have been making breathing more effortful.

Of course, you'll need to "drop into" felt experience without an agenda or plan, without expectations, and without interpretive thinking if you want to reach a more restorative state of breathing and ESA. The result could be a relaxation of all the muscles in the body, a felt sense of safety and trust in the not-knowing, and a totally relaxed breath with a long expiratory pause. This may not be so easy to accomplish in a busy airport, but with practice, restorative ESA can find us almost anywhere.

You might have a TPN-based insight that your breath becomes constricted because as a child your wishes were rarely granted and you are still waiting—holding your breath—for something good to happen. That is a helpful insight about your own vulnerabilities, one that will potentially help you sustain a modulated ESA state. But unless your breath and body spontaneously relax with this insight—even though it is pointing to something that may have been the case for you—the insight alone is not going to put an end to your breath holding. You'll have to go deeper into your felt experience of waiting and wanting, of not being seen or heard, of disappointment, grief, and anger. For this, you need to give yourself plenty of space for patience and practice, or find a therapist who can guide you through learning to modulate your challenging memories and emotions and perhaps into the vastness and peace of restoration.

Restorative ESA, going into your felt experience in the present moment, is always heralded by the onset of a relaxed breathing pattern. And this is partly why restorative ESA is so conducive to health and well-being. A relaxed breath improves blood flow and oxygenation, promotes the cleansing of toxic stress hormones, enhances immune function, eases muscle tension, and allows us the felt sense of safety and the permission to let go of thinking and doing.

Summary and Conclusions

In this chapter the experiences of pain, eating, and breathing—and how they change as we move between different states of ESA—are offered as examples of the themes of this book as manifested in everyday life. As in the previous chapter, the take-home message is *not* that you have to be in a state of restorative ESA all the time. You can't be. It is impossible to stay there and still live a reasonably active and productive life.

The take-home message, one that we all have the ability to use on a daily basis, is to continue to cultivate our present-moment awareness of our state of ESA. All the examples in this, previous, and subsequent chapters are given to assist you in noticing in which state you happen to be living at any moment. Identifying your current state and noticing when you are shifting states allow for the possibility to make a choice to shift into a more modulated or restorative state and give you a growing sense of self-confidence in your ability to track your own changes.

This confidence may be hard-earned. You may need a lot of practice. You may need a lot of support and guidance, especially if you tend to get easily dysregulated and find yourself unable to make the shift into modulated states.

Building your embodied self-awareness is like learning any form of body-based activity, such as dance, music, or athletics. Remember that the conduction pathways for felt experiences—like interoception and proprioception from the body's periphery to the brain—are slow, clunky, fuzzy, and hard to get ahold of; we can easily get lost and frustrated in the process. Well, that just *is* the process, so give yourself a break, do what you can today, and start again tomorrow.

It takes a toddler more than a year to learn to walk with stability and confidence, and there are many falls along the way. It takes at least three to five years to learn to speak a first language in reasonably coherent sentences with reasonably clear pronunciation, and those are only the baby steps of language use. Taking the steps—one at a time and over a long period of time, feeling your way through the process—is the only way to grow in your nervous system a more finely tuned ability to walk the walk and talk the talk of your own embodied self-awareness.

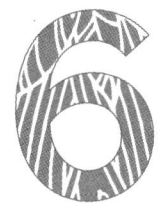

How Our State of Embodied Self-Awareness Affects Emotional Experiences

Emotions are often classified as either positive or negative. Enjoyment, excitement, or love might be a positive emotion, while a negative emotion might be sadness, anger, or fear. In line with the theme of this book, this chapter will propose that the division between positive and negative emotions is misleading. Each emotion is an essential ingredient of a full human experience. This book makes the case that a more useful distinction than positive/negative is how each emotion may be experienced: as restorative, modulated, or dysregulated.

Dysregulated enjoyment? What about addiction and perverse sadism? Modulated fear? What about flow and eustress that bring us to the edge of our abilities—jumping off a cliff for hang gliding, or surfing gigantic and dangerous waves—but still let us be in control? Restorative anger? What about feelings of empowerment, justice, and inner strength that are not directed toward harm or blame of others?

Not everyone agrees that emotions are a fundamental and essential part of human experience. Researchers from the Department of Psychological Sciences at the University of California, Irvine (USA), discovered that people have different beliefs about whether emotional feelings are helpful or unhelpful in their lives. People in the group believing that emotions are helpful said that emotions—all the emotions—are important sources of information about their lives and choices; emotions contributed to their sense of wisdom and personal strength. People in the unhelpful group thought emotions are a form of human weakness—distracting causes of confusion that interfere with making rational choices.[1]

The people who found emotions helpful, however, reported greater well-being, emotional acceptance, and the use of emotional intelligence to modulate emotion. People in this group showed greater physiological reactivity while viewing a distressing film, and they were more accepting of their emotional response compared to people in the emotions-are-unhelpful group. After watching the film, the people in the helpful group showed more decrease in arousal and were less likely to suppress their feelings, which returned to normal after a short period. The people in the unhelpful group reported less well-being, greater emotional suppression, and more substance use. In the language of this book, the emotions-are-helpful group could be interpreted as feeling their emotions in more modulated and restorative states, while the people in the other group are more accustomed to experiencing emotion in a dysregulated manner.

Research done at the University of Utrecht (the Netherlands) on 403 women with fibromyalgia and 126 women with no such symptoms found that emotional suppression was significantly more likely in the fibromyalgia group. The authors concluded,

When negative emotions are approached by acknowledging, expressing, and reappraising them, resolution may occur by habituation, development of insight, strengthening of social support, and improved self-regulation. On the other hand, when individuals lack emotional awareness or suppress or otherwise avoid their emotions, repeated emotional intrusions and elevated physiological arousal occur, which may eventuate in heightened susceptibility to somatic disturbances and the experience of physical symptoms.[2]

Beliefs that emotions are not helpful, and the subsequent tendency to experience emotions as dysregulated and as needing to be suppressed, can be a factor in the formation of inflammation and disease states. On the other hand, people who are able to feel and express a wider variety of emotions have lower biomarkers of inflammation, which makes them less susceptible to chronic illnesses such as fibromyalgia and dysfunction of gastrointestinal, cardiovascular, and immune systems.[3]

Similarly, people who are more able to express their grief after the loss of a spouse have lower levels of inflammation compared to those who try to suppress their emotions.[4] Each state of embodied self-awareness (ESA) is a synergistic connection between all felt experiences, types of thinking, and autonomic nervous system functions that regulate all the systems of the body that both maintain health and promote illness.

An example of this synergy is an observed link between interoception and proprioception with emotional awareness. Research done at the Department of Psychology, University of California, Berkeley (USA), shows higher levels of emotional awareness in vipassana meditators who practice attention to felt experiences in the body and dancers who are trained especially in proprioceptive awareness of the felt sense of the body in motion, compared to people who are not trained in any embodied practice.[5] This link is likely due to the fact that interoceptive feelings related to emotions, such as heart rate, overlap in the anterior insula with emotional evaluations.[6]

As mentioned earlier in this book, interoceptive, proprioceptive, and autonomic feelings (see Table 1.2, p. 11) rarely occur without some kind of emotional evaluation. Felt experience is almost always combined with the emotional tone of feeling good or bad, wanted or unwanted, something to approach or something to avoid. Emotions, in other words, provide a kind of "color" or "flavor" to every felt experience, helping us make choices to feel or not to feel some sensation.

Modulated and restorative ESA are states in which we use different kinds of strategies to stay with difficult feelings—such as pain, or hatred, or disgust—that our body wants to avoid. In modulated states, we can use our TPN (task-positive network) thinking in the form of emotional intelligence to stay focused on an unpleasant feeling long enough to identify it, manage it, understand where it is coming from, and explain it to ourselves. This modulatory control keeps our emotions in tolerable bounds using sympathetic arousal. The overlap of emotional and interoceptive information in the anterior insula not only enhances our felt experience but also assists in the TPN interpretive process, providing us with cognitive coping strategies and self-talk that allow us to be more effective in modulating the emotional experience.[7]

A research study done at the School of Nursing at the University of Washington (Seattle, USA) explored a clinical intervention that helped people use modulated ESA—via both brief access to felt experience and TPN explanations—to cope with emotions. One client from the study, a forty-year-old woman with chronic back pain, was asked by her therapist to feel the achiness in her back. As she explored the interoceptive pain, an emotion started to arise.

> *She feels her throat tighten and tears come to her eyes. The therapist asks what she is noticing, and she says "I just feel so sad," crying quietly with her eyes closed. The client explains that she is remembering her brother who died 2 years ago and that she's not had a chance to really mourn: "I feel like I just need to cry and let him go. I miss him so much."*[8]

The pain in her back began to lessen, and the client reported that she was not aware of how she was holding back the emotion of sadness. She was accessing the grief, perhaps for the first time, while at the same time trying to make sense of where it came from in her thought process.

> *[The client] says, "I feel like I've been doing my best to just keep going after he died. But I think I just didn't want to feel how bad it hurt to have him gone." She reflects further on when her pain started and continues: "I've been trying my best to ignore my back pain and here I am remembering my brother and how much I miss him." She wonders out loud about whether her avoidant coping style may further distance her from knowing how she feels about aspects of her life.*[9]

This example illustrates this link between interoception, emotion, and modulated TPN thinking. There is a clear combination of some brief moments of felt experience—both the interoception of back pain and the emotion of sadness—along with the client's TPN interpretations and her attempts to understand how her back pain is related to her brother's death. And clearly, naming and interpreting emotional experiences during modulated states can provide at least a temporary respite from not only physical pain but also emotional pain.[10]

In this client, and in all of us, there is still an opportunity to shift from modulation to restoration. In restorative states we simply surrender to the feeling of sadness and grief (or whatever is there). We allow it to arise and be felt with no effort to understand, interpret, or modulate it. The result, as we have seen, is usually that the emotional feeling builds, peaks, and then subsides into a felt sense of relief and parasympathetic relaxation. The client in this research study did not get to this place. Continuing to revisit the feeling in small doses may eventually lead her into restorative, parasympathetic states that may engender a reduction and perhaps complete absence of the tension in the tight muscles contributing to her back pain.

It seems easy, doesn't it? If we just let ourselves feel our emotions and not try to figure things out, we'll be rewarded with peace, healing, and contentment. Something long-suppressed and hidden can come to the surface, and we are finally relieved of a traumatic burden. If we are in a dysregulated pattern, however, this does not seem easy at all. We may have a deep-seated fear and accompanying ruminative thoughts that the emotion will consume us, that we have to do everything in our power to suppress it, to hold back our tears of rage or even joy.[11] If we can modulate, as in the back-pain example, we can get a little closer to the emotion and the pain, but the most likely outcome is that the pain will return, with or without the feeling of grief.

Restorative emotions happen when we let down our guard, when we let our emotions arise spontaneously. As we have learned in this book, it is not so easy to get to this state. It takes practice, guidance, support, and a sense of total safety and security. Restorative emotions can't happen when we stop the process of felt experience in order to explain it to ourselves. We have to notice those thoughts and let them go as we surrender to wherever the emotion may take us. In addition to the combination of interoception and emotion in the anterior insula, activation of the ventromedial prefrontal cortex is also involved in this ability to access restorative states of more deeply felt emotion.[12]

The theme of this chapter is to describe the felt experience of different emotions in each of the three states of embodied self-awareness (ESA). These descriptions may provide some support for gaining the courage to fall into the unknown of letting ourselves feel emotions in a way that leads to whole-body healing and restoration.

Anger/Rage

Anger is one of the primary human emotions. It has an adaptive significance that evolved over millennia as a way of defending ourselves when someone or something is getting in our way, interrupting something we are doing, or holding us back from completing a goal. Anger also occurs when our bodies, our expressions, or our words are attacked, threatened, or wounded. Anger is a possible response to pain, to betrayal, to abandonment, to loss of something that we considered ours.

Dysregulated ESA of Anger

Anger becomes dysregulated when we cannot find the means to safely feel and metabolize it, or when our means of regulation becomes insufficient to keep our actions in check. Dysregulated anger (fight) takes the form of acting out, rebellion, hostility, violence, malice, threatening, glaring, looming, intimidating, hurting, killing, abusing, or assaulting. It can also take the form of depression as anger is shut down and turned inward, a sense of paralysis, or passive-aggressive behavior (freeze).

The specific form of dysregulated anger depends on the social-interpersonal circumstances as well as the possible presence of illness and pain conditions in the body. If one lives in a society or culture where attack, counterattack, betrayal, and retribution are part of the fabric of life, then dysregulated anger is going to be more overt and possibly violent. In subcultures with norms that foment and perpetuate hatred, terrorism, intertribal or ethnic warfare, gangs, discrimination, rape, honor killings, or domestic abuse, dysregulated anger may even be considered socially acceptable.

Some forms of dysregulated anger result from stress and trauma. If we were hurt or attacked in a situation that was dangerous, in which we were alone and unable to defend ourselves—as in child or adult assault and sexual abuse—dysregulated anger may be transformed into acting out, becoming a bully, or abusing others; it could also become paralysis, suppression, denial, becoming a victim, or giving up.

Research done at the Department of Psychology, Rosalind Franklin University of Medicine and Science (Chicago, Illinois, USA), shows that feelings of dysregulated anger may also be connected to chronic pain conditions. In people with chronic low-back pain, for example, increased tension in the muscles of the lower back was correlated with high levels of expressed and felt anger. This effect appears to be mediated by an amygdala-based stress reaction that alters the connections between the insula and the anterior cingulate cortex[13] (some of the brain centers for emotional felt experience; see Figure 2.5, p. 68).

When we are in pain (see chapter 5, p. 139) or suffering from any chronic illness, we are more likely to lash out at others for no apparent reason. Dysregulated pain and the attempts to avoid feeling it make it more likely that we will try to escape the feeling by lashing out. In fact, research done at Keele and Oxford Universities (UK) shows that swearing can actually reduce the felt experience of pain. In the study, they measured several self-report questionnaires and physiological indicators of pain when people were asked—in response to a laboratory-induced painful stimulation—to repeat the common swear word *fuck*, compared with made-up words that sounded like swear words, such as *fouch*.

The made-up words had absolutely no effect on pain levels, whereas *fuck* was indeed effective in pain reduction.[14] This is a clear example of how the fight response during dysregulation (see chapter 3, p. 75)—in this case, yelling a swear word as if to get the pain out of the body—works at least for a short time to escape from felt experience. But like all dysregulated emotions, this strategy is short-lived, and the end result is being stuck in a state of persistent pain, anger, and irritability.

Thoughts about dysregulated anger may be ruminative, self-focused, and self-justifying, including thoughts about injustice, blaming, hatred, judgment, or resentment. These thoughts and the dysregulated anger can lead to domestic violence, terrorism, and hatred of and attacks against people of different races, ethnicities, or gender orientations. The long history of violence against children, women, people of color, Jews, and many other religious minorities is likely fueled by a sense of dysregulated resentment that is passed from one generation to the next.

We may be always on edge, ready to pounce on anyone or anything. We may say negative or hurtful things or want to wound someone physically or emotionally. We may use anger to cheat or lie or feel justified to take and use anything. We can sometimes boil over in a fit of rage and can't control it. We easily can reach a breaking point physically and emotionally. Dysregulated angry thoughts can also be directed toward the self in the form of shame, inadequacy, self-harm, guilt, or self-blame.

We are completely out of touch with the possibility of facing these painful feelings that may trigger the anger and that we need to feel in order to break out of this dysregulated state. Engaging with these feelings provides the possibility of bringing ourselves to a place where we can truly own and acknowledge how we have been hurt by what may have been done to us.

Modulated ESA of Anger

In modulated ESA there can be the same kinds of angry feelings as in dysregulated ESA: impatience, frustration, self- and other-blame, revenge, irritability, or resentment. Modulation of these feelings is accomplished by active self-control over our actions, such as pushing ourselves to get past these feelings, not wanting to talk about them, focusing on "good" things, trying to forget, and using other cognitive-behavioral strategies of inner speech. Alternatively, we can decide to discuss these feelings with another person in a way that may lead to compromise and negotiation, an agreement to move on, or possibly forgiveness: verbal and communicative strategies for self-modulation.

A collaborative study done at Eindhoven University of Technology (the Netherlands) and the Leeds School of Business at the University of Colorado (Boulder, USA) examined how employees at a large corporation handled everyday stressors on the job. Those employees who exhibited "sportsmanship," defined as a willingness to tolerate the annoyances at work (such as distractions, discomforts, or demands) without complaining were better able to modulate their initial feelings of disappointment and anger. They were more able to calm themselves and feel better about themselves compared to employees who had a shorter fuse, who were more likely to show irritation and to complain.[15]

On the other hand, like all emotional intelligence strategies for modulation, these effects are likely to be short-term because being a good sport gets old fast if the work environment does not improve. Another step in a more lasting modulated emotional intelligence strategy is to find a way to talk with supervisors and fellow employees about the discomfort and anger. Many organizational environments, however, are not open to employees' feedback, most especially when the organization maintains a culture of sexual or verbal harassment, retaliation and intimidation of employees, or other negative or dismissive leadership styles. Whistleblowers in these environments are genuinely at risk of losing their jobs, which sustains the toxic culture of the workplace and forces employees to continually modulate until they "lose it" in a dysregulated outburst and/or get fired or quit.

Workplaces and other environments that encourage sharing emotions and listening to complaints and concerns have a greater employee sense of belonging and feeling heard and fewer overtly expressed angry responses.[16] This means that how we modulate difficult emotions—any emotions, in fact—is often not up to the individual but a direct consequence of the social-relational environment.

Using mindfulness strategies is another way to modulate anger. According to Jessica Morey, executive director of Inward Bound Mindfulness Education,

> *Anger is a natural, life-affirming emotion. It lets us know when a boundary has been crossed, when our needs are not being met, or when someone we care about is in danger. Being mindful of anger means not suppressing, denying or avoiding it and also not acting out in harmful ways. Instead, connect with the direct experience of the anger, and then decide what action you want to take.*[17]

This act of decision making is what makes this a modulated strategy. In modulated ESA we can say, "I'm angry," or we can think or talk about how someone or something made us feel angry and why we might feel angry. We might think about what to do or say, who might be at fault and why. We can talk ourselves into feeling more angry or less angry. We can share these thoughts with others. We can help organize protests or campaigns that seek to restore justice.

As the embodied feeling of being angry begins to form, our thoughts come in to keep us from moving too deeply into the feeling of what *we think* is going to be intolerable, what *we think* may lead to doing something we would regret. Our thoughts and postures are keeping the lid on our feelings of anger, keeping the anger in this modulated state: just under the surface, with or without a resolution. At the same time, we continue to believe that the way to resolve these feelings is by intentional problem solving, which keeps us in a modulated sympathetic state of thinking, deciding, and doing.

Restorative ESA of Anger

There is a way that a potentially toxic emotion such as anger can not only be modulated but may also be restorative. As for all forms of restoration, this requires us to let go of control, stop thinking and explaining, and just sit in the felt experience. Anger easily bursts out of us, so feeling the anger in stillness—without the need to react to it or do anything about it—is not a particularly easy path.

For wounds that are the most intense, learning to tolerate and talk about these feelings in modulated ESA is an important transitional step, one that may take years and lots of help from other people, most likely trained therapists and ESA practitioners. Entering restorative anger states, we also have to tolerate feeling how the anger has taken a toll on our body and relationships, and perhaps how—when dysregulated—we may have hurt ourselves and blameless others. Anger is perhaps the most toxic emotion in the sense that it invades the body like a virus and resists our attempts to come to terms with it.

Anger is restorative only if we can fully feel the immensity of it without acting it out or holding on to the tension of hatred or revenge. Anger, however intense, is just a feeling, and like all feelings, once we allow them to be felt, they will pass. All forms of restorative emotion have a natural onset, a rise in intensity, and a decline in our awareness and expression that is accompanied by a felt sense of "recovery," "coming down," and "completeness" as the body moves into parasympathetic relaxation. This is part of the healing power of restorative ESA: as we learn to trust in letting go of control and allowing our real feelings to emerge, our nervous system will lead the way in the process of supporting all other body systems to metabolize the emotion and come to rest.

When an anger episode starts, we may begin to sense a burning in the arms and hands and the very alive feeling of wanting to strike out at someone, and we just let the feeling arise. Or we may feel a tightness in the gut and let that be there as it grows into an almost unbearable pain and transforms into feelings like shame and defeat and a memory of not being able to defend ourselves. We may feel how the body was torn apart by an accident, surgery, abandonment, or assault, or maybe intense hatred toward others—particular others or members of a group deemed to be inferior and worthy of disdain, or who may have hurt or killed people like us or members of our family—and a building urge to retaliate or get revenge. Or we feel a constriction around the eyes and jaw and mouth, and the very real urge to shout obscenities or hurtful words, and we can let those feelings expand into a sense of our own power and ability to take care of ourselves. In this way, restorative anger can come to feel empowering.

The restorative experience of anger can thus transform into feelings of inner strength, personal power, and passion. These feelings do not need an outward retaliation: they are filled with a sense of our own integrity, of the possibility of standing up for ourselves in the future. It can feel like coming through a battle victorious, the battle having been waged within the self to confront and subdue the seething demon within and the memories of surviving having been hurt by others.

And in all these cases, these deeper feelings morph into a parasympathetic relief as if the body "gets it," a "yes," that is how we felt, that's what we suffered, and we don't need to hold on to that unrequited rage anymore. Restorative experiences of anger may take many repetitions of this sequence and a long period of time for the body to fully metabolize the toxicity and for the ultimate emergence of our own strength to stand in the center of the storm.

Fear/Anxiety

Fear or anxiety is also a primary emotion that can occur whenever we sense threat. This could be threat from the outside, including some of the same situations mentioned for anger. It could also be a felt sense of threat from inside of our body including pain, illness, and discomfort.

Dysregulated ESA of Fear

One of the more common forms of dysregulated anxiety, called *generalized anxiety disorder*, is related to the same kinds of alterations in neurophysiology that are seen in all types of dysregulated states. A group of psychiatrists and behavioral medicine specialists at George Washington University (Washington, DC, USA) writes that:

> *Anxiety can create excessive sympathetic activation, alteration in inflammatory response, and disruption of the hypothalamic-pituitary-adrenal axis—predisposing patients to increased health risks. [The combination of] anxiety disorders and medical illnesses often lead to a self-perpetuating cycle in which a chronic medical illness negatively affects level of function, leading to depression and anxiety, which, in turn, can worsen the underlying medical condition. Patients with primary anxiety disorders are more likely to suffer from GI, respiratory, cardiac, and neurological disorders, even after adjusting for confounding factors such as sex, depression, and substance use disorders.[18]*

People who suffer from generalized anxiety disorder related to past stress and trauma are more likely to show higher co-activation of the amygdala and insula, bypassing the modulatory effects of the medial prefrontal cortex.[19] If this condition continues without treatment, it can lead to symptomatic depression, anxiety, paranoia, dissociative identities, suicidal thoughts, and so on. A racing heart, for example, can create a dysregulated state of high anxiety while suppressing other felt experiences such as pain.[20]

The physiological manifestations of anxiety show up in many different life situations. Waiting to go onstage prior to a performance, music students who reported higher levels of anxiety had greater variability in breathing patterns compared to more confident students. Disturbances in breathing (see chapter 5, p. 167) are common symptoms of fear, panic, and anxiety. The anxious students sometimes took deep breaths, sometimes short and shallow breaths, and they showed a higher rate of troubled sighing.[21]

The most salient felt experiences of dysregulated fear/anxiety, therefore, are an inability to breathe, constriction in the throat and chest, tremors, postural instability, hyperventilation, and dizziness. We can use our fight response by gasping for breath or our flight response by wanting to run or hide. We can become completely frozen and helpless, which occurs when dorsal vagal "immobilization with fear" pathways lead to paralysis, the inability to react or cry out, lack of clear thoughts, and feelings of confusion, disorientation, numbness, blackout, or total aloneness and alienation.

There may also be ruminative and catastrophizing thoughts: "I'm going to die, I need to scream for help but no sound comes, I can't escape, I have to run away but where do I go?" In anxiety, the words feel caught in the throat where the air can't go in or out except for gasping, which leads to more thoughts of desperation and feelings of claustrophobia and tightness.

In these panic states, we may, in fact, never actually feel the fear. In our rush to bury it, push it away, give in to addictions or immobility, the fear underneath never is able to be felt, never finds comfort, and lies in wait for the next episode, the next attack, about which we have a nagging feeling of worry related to our inability to modulate the next experience. A real panic attack is traumatic, which sets up the fear pathways in the nervous system (amygdala and hypothalamus for ANS activation, and hippocampus for remembering fearful situations) to be even more sensitive to another episode of anxiety and panic, one we think that we can never fully recover from.[22]

Modulated ESA of Fear

In modulated fear, we have more of a sense of control over, and thus more ability to access, our felt experience of being afraid. We may be able to allow ourselves to feel restless, anxious, jumpy, uncertain, lost, or unable to stay grounded, along with the urge to move, run, or hide. We may feel momentarily paralyzed in our thoughts or actions. If what caused the fear is brief—like a loud noise or a near-miss accident—we can more easily feel our breath get short, our muscles tighten, our hands shake, and we can more easily settle ourselves with thoughts ("Nothing serious. I'm OK. Just breathe.") and let the fear dissipate as we return to normal activity. In these brief fearful moments, we may be able to connect with the feeling of fear and then continue with our activity. We can drink some water, get a hug, walk it off, shake it out.

With something more threatening—an ongoing work or family relationship that feels threatening, a likely attack, or the present situation evoking a body memory of trauma—we may have a felt experience of a tightening in the muscles around the trachea, setting off the air-hunger receptors and creating a feeling of being choked or strangled. At the same time, the muscles in the neck, upper chest, and shoulders begin to contract to pull up the rib cage to get more air into the lungs because the diaphragm is tight from the sense of danger coming from the body, constricting chest expansion from below. Possibly the abdominal-wall muscles and gut contract with feelings of nausea, burping, gas, distension, pain—all brewing in the background as attention is directed to the upper chest and chest walls trying to expand but beginning to freeze up. Then the jaw tightens and the vagus nerve's pathways in the face, ears, throat, and skull begin to create a feeling of the head being crushed.

Modulated fear means that we can attempt to manage these feelings using TPN thinking: "I'm going to be OK, just slow down, feel my feet, take some deep breaths, get up and move." Or we might do something we know that eases the growing panic, such as drinking a cup of tea, going for a walk, talking to someone, taking our anxiety medication, doing yoga or controlled breathing exercises, meditating, seeing a therapist, and so forth.

In her published meditation journal, Mary Booker, a drama therapist from the UK, describes doing a meditative movement practice on the porch of a temple on the island of Java in Indonesia. The practice was meant to connect the person with the environment of the surrounding jungle.

While doing movement practice at Sukha Temple, some very large bees arrived: Standing still. Breathing. The bees come very close, curious, insistent. To my face, eyes, ears. I feel the wind of their wings. Many times over the day! Really feeling how hard it is to stay still in fear.[23]

By using this kind of mindfulness about our felt experience of fearful things, if we succeed in helping the immediate panic to dissipate, we can begin to feel more "normal" and return to what we were doing. We get back to work or our meditative movement; we show up.

We might want to talk about the fear with another person: "I got really scared in the situation earlier." "Noisy social gatherings make me feel nervous, and it's like I don't know what to do with myself." "Working out at the gym makes me anxious because I feel like people are looking at my body and judging me." These kinds of honest self-descriptions help us modulate the experience, and hearing feedback from others could help in managing the next such situation.

Restorative ESA of Fear

Actually feeling fear without having to do something about it (meaning that we just feel and do not engage any of the modulatory strategies mentioned earlier) requires a sense of safety and support, usually with another person who can help us stay present with the feeling. Actually feeling fear may mean letting our body shake uncontrollably.[24] This happens when we let go of the muscle tension, especially in the gut and diaphragm, that we have been using in an attempt to contain and modulate the fear. Actually feeling fear may mean we experience a full-blown panic attack: shortness of breath, the urge to run or fight, to get away from the claustrophobic enclosure of our chest and throat getting tighter and tighter.

Actually feeling the fear means allowing all these feelings to completely take us to the point where it may seem as if we are going to die, or vomit, or cough uncontrollably; there might be lip tremors, palpitations, shaking, and aches in the chest where the muscles were strained.

We may be able to allow authentically felt panic: the deep cosmic fear of death, of the end, of the edge of the abyss, how close we came to the uncontrollable pull of annihilation. Allowing all this can awaken some deeper sense of loss or hopelessness or despair that the cause of the fear will never end. And this feeling under the fear, the "truth" of it, somehow brings a sense of relief. The parasympathetic nervous system allows the breath to come in, the tension to ease, and the "real" underlying feelings that may have triggered the fear to emerge in awareness.

As this happens, we gain the possibility of recovery as the body begins to ease into a partial parasympathetic response, as more oxygen begins to wake up parts of the brain that had been shut down. There is more mental and visual clarity as the ears are opening up to the sounds around. The internal muscles of the ears and eyes begin to soften with parasympathetic vagal activation.

Then there may come a shudder of the whole body, and another, sweetening into a gentle tremor with a tingling feeling returning to the limbs. There is a gradually spreading feeling of warmth and softness, gratitude and maybe sobs convulsing into releases bringing large gulps of oxygen and resonant thoughts—"I made it, I'm still here, I'm really OK now, I survived"—and maybe gut relaxation noises.

Actually feeling fear may mean that as the tension begins to ease in this way, the body suddenly remembers the old traumatic threat, and the panic returns with its full force of suffocation. Once again, if we have a feeling of safety and support in the present moment, we can ride this all the way into almost disappearing, until we once again discover a powerful and real feeling "under" the fear that opens up and expands our lungs and brings relief.

Actually feeling the fear is likely to bring multiple waves of panic, but each time we can go through this cycle of panic and relief, the panic becomes less intense, the episodes are shorter in duration, and we become less afraid of feeling panic because our body is learning that panic is just a feeling and will not last forever, that it will end, and that we will feel better for not fighting the feeling, not trying to hold it back but letting it take us to the point where we can find a deeper meaning and truth about what happened in the past. At this point, the relief and aching in the chest and soreness in the face and neck are a reminder of being still alive and capable of feeling, which brings perhaps more gasps and sobs, and the cycle repeats—perhaps many times—until it is finally over and the panic attacks and their aftereffects have completely dissipated.

Enjoyment/Pleasure

Enjoyment is a basic emotion that is revealed in many different forms and expressions. The emotional expression most typically associated with enjoyment—smiling—is not always associated with pleasure. Genuine smiles of enjoyment are so-called felt smiles. They involve the full face with a raising of the cheeks and a crinkling around the eye corners. Felt smiles occur in engaging, enjoyable, and humorous situations. They are symmetrical and often go with bright eyes, body movements reflecting happiness, and sounds like laughter, crying, or words expressing joy.

So-called false smiles, on the other hand, involve primarily the mouth, with lip corners upturned, but not the rest of the face. The lips are usually pressed and the smile is slightly asymmetrical. False smiles occur in social situations where one is required to be polite or submissive. These are smiles we give in elevators, when we meet a stranger's gaze on a sidewalk, or when confronted by a demanding boss. False smiles are intended to hide difficult feelings such as discomfort, shame, or anger and are clearly not reflecting feelings of enjoyment.

Finally, so-called miserable smiles—unlike false smiles—do not attempt to hide negative feelings. They typically occur along with expressions of distress, disgust, or sadness. Miserable smiles reveal the person's true feelings but give the impression to others that those feelings are modulated. It is as if the person is saying, nonverbally, "I feel bad but I'm really OK."[25]

Conversely, just as smiles may reflect emotions other than enjoyment, the experience of "felt" or genuine enjoyment is not reflected in a single emotional expression. It can take many forms, from laughter to crying (tears of joy), from aroused excitement to simple pleasure. Restorative enjoyment brings a sense of peace and relaxation, while dysregulated enjoyment can feel compulsive and potentially harmful and may include facial expressions with malicious intent such as sneering, leering, or disdain.

A questionnaire study was done at the Mental Health Research Unit of Kingsway Hospital (Derby, UK) on 203 undergraduate students from the University of Derby. The students had an age range from eighteen to fifty-six, with an average age of twenty-three. The study found that these students reported three different types of positive emotion. The first was what they called "Active," which consists of feeling lively, energetic, excited, enthusiastic, adventurous, dynamic, and eager. The second form of positive emotion was called "Relaxed," which includes feeling calm, peaceful, tranquil, laid back, and serene. The final form was called "Safe/Content," with feelings of safety, security, contentment, and warmth.

Students reporting either Relaxed or Safe/Content feelings scored lower on overall stress levels. On the other hand, only the students who reported more of the Safe/Content emotion scored lower on measures of anxiety, depression, and self-criticism and higher on measures of self-assurance and ability to get close to other people. Those who had the highest scores on Active positive emotion showed no consistent pattern of relationship either to positive or negative outcomes.

This study suggests that only the positive emotion of Safe/Content serves as a protective factor against forms of dysregulated ESA because the feelings of safety, security, and contentment are most clearly connected with multiple types of restoration. Active and Relaxed forms of positive emotion, on the other hand, are most likely part of being in a state of sympathetically aroused modulated ESA.[26]

Another, similar study at Arizona State University (Tempe, USA) examined physiological reactions to the following positive emotions: anticipatory enthusiasm, attachment love, nurturant love, amusement, and awe. Only awe was consistently associated with a sustained parasympathetic relaxation response reflective of restorative ESA. All the other forms of positive emotion in the study showed at least some sympathetic activation and were therefore part of a state of modulated ESA.[27]

Dysregulated ESA of Enjoyment

If we are dysregulated, we may believe that addiction, risk taking, lashing out, being manic, or having an out-of-body and altered-state experience is enjoyable. This is because these methods have the effect of temporarily numbing our pain. The rush of a drug, the loosening of alcohol, the thrill of driving fast and road rage, the illusory sense of power from hurting another person or nonconsensual sexual sadism, abuse, or harassment, the tuning out of reality with dissociative states: these all may seem perversely enjoyable.[28] If we have been habitually dysregulated because of a history of trauma, this may be the only way we have ever experienced anything like pleasure.

All of these states, however, do not lead to ventral vagal parasympathetic restoration. Instead, there is a high level of arousal (or pain), fear, anger, loss, or trauma that is not felt and certainly not modulated.

Modulated ESA of Enjoyment

The sense of modulated enjoyment is primarily during a state of sympathetic arousal—being excited, "up," intense, focused, and engaged. This state can be rewarding, but it is not, in itself, restorative because parasympathetic moments are brief. It is more like a refreshing shower than a long soothing bath. This type of enjoyment comes during "flow" states where we are at the edge of our abilities—in sports, debate, conversation, business transactions, creative work, performing arts, and so on—sympathetically aroused yet attuned and in control (see chapter 3, p. 94).

A more modest, less aroused form of modulated enjoyment may also occur. This can happen when we share smiles and laughs with other people. It can also be a moment of mild amusement at hearing a comment or a joke that is only sort of funny. Or it could be moments of playing with a child or friend when, what was just a moment ago a really enjoyable exchange, shifts in intent as the other person becomes more playfully aggressive in a way that makes us somewhat amused and somewhat uncomfortable.

Modulated enjoyment is often brief and part of another ongoing process, such as a good laugh that punctuates an otherwise serious conversation. Laughter during conversation actually makes it easier for people to talk about themselves in narrative (TPN) language,[29] enhancing the state of modulated ESA. Stand-up comedians—the best ones, at least—are very good at using modulated strategies to elicit certain types of laughter at particular times from an audience. Usually jokes that get the biggest laughs come at the opening of the performance, followed by the comedian's deliberate pacing for the remainder of the show, during which smaller laughs are more likely to occur.[30] The audience, on the other hand, is sympathetically

aroused, using focused modulated attention and rapt listening to the mono-
logue. This focused attention of the audience, which is created by the performer, means that sympathetic activation is likely to persist even during the
laughing episodes.

One can be enjoying eating something delicious while reading, checking email, talking, or having a lot of thoughts. The pleasurable tastes are
present but often modulated by wanting to get back to the other ongoing
activities (recall the Chocolate Decadence example, p. 162). The same can
be true of any seemingly pleasurable activity like exercise, yoga, resting,
being in nature, or being with people we love: we take in only small bits of
enjoyment that our modulatory process—which is keeping track of our lives,
staying plugged in, and filling our thoughts—permits us to have.

Modulated enjoyment can also co-occur with the engagement of the
TPN. Research conducted at Case Western Reserve University (Cleveland,
Ohio, USA) showed that this co-occurrence was effective in leadership teams
in work organizations. People who were able to enact both enjoyment and
problem-solving strategies at work were better able to build collaborative
teams that could develop creative visions for the future and create opportunities for career advancement.[31]

Restorative ESA of Enjoyment

Happiness is like a butterfly which, when pursued, is always beyond our
grasp, but, if you will sit down quietly, may alight upon you.

—ANONYMOUS, FROM VARIOUS SOURCES IN THE LATE 1840s

This quote, which is sometimes but incorrectly attributed to Nathaniel
Hawthorne, reflects the nature of restorative enjoyment. Unlike modulated
enjoyment in which we are doing something to have fun or to be funny—in
which there is sympathetic effort—restorative enjoyment, like all restorative
felt experiences, is something that "alights," or arrives in us without effort.

Restorative enjoyment can take many forms including the felt experience
of relaxation when we are able to let go of our muscular tension/armoring,
a warm and spreading sense of relief, feelings of recovering and healing, of

feeling soothed, safe, blessed, hopeful, settled, filled up and complete, vulnerable, open, content, peaceful, fully present, and alive.

With other people, restorative enjoyment can involve feelings of total acceptance, surrender, safety, deep states of connection, love, appreciation, being seen or held, compassion, shared warmth, melting, softening, and receptivity. Enjoyment related to interpersonal physical connection, closeness, and empathy has restorative effects on health such as a lowering of heart rate and an increase of parasympathetic activation.[32]

These forms of restorative enjoyment typically stabilize heart rhythms that create feedback to the brain that triggers a sustained parasympathetic relaxation and dorsal vagal immobilization without fear: how good it can feel to stop all the activity and just come into the present moment.[33] This kind of enjoyment is softer and sweeter than modulated enjoyment. Instead of modulated laughter, celebration, dancing, and fist pumping, for example, restorative enjoyment may be revealed by a softening of facial expressions, a more youthful appearance in the face, or a gentle smile with bright eyes.

As a prelude to the next section on sadness, listening to "sad" music can often evoke restorative enjoyment in the form of feelings of compassion and empathy, the kind of joy that may bring tears and the feeling of being touched, according to researchers at Ohio State University (Columbus, USA) and the University of Oslo (Norway).[34] In the 1940s, German philosopher Helmuth Plessner wrote that crying of this sort may occur "before the sublimity of a work of art or a landscape … the touching candor and familiarity of children … in situations where the attempt to 'do something' no longer arises. Essential for the onset of tears on such occasions is the sudden transition from an attitude of tension to one of relaxation."[35]

Sadness/Grief

The most typical form of sadness expression is crying. As we just saw, however, crying can also express relieved happiness. Sometimes it is difficult to disentangle the different emotions that may be involved in crying. Generally speaking, and again in the words of Helmuth Plessner, sadness-related crying occurs "when we become aware of a superior force against which we can do nothing,"[36] such as emotional and physical pain, loss, separation, or an external force of aggression—all of which connect crying with our inability to change or resist these forces.

Dysregulated ESA of Sadness

As usual, one of the hallmarks of dysregulated felt experience is the active suppression of the feeling and its expression. In the case of sadness, loss, or grief, suppression of crying can have adverse health effects brought about by increased sympathetic activation needed to stop ourselves from crying and the loss of the ability to release held muscle tension in the body.[37] Crying may be suppressed in front of a group of people when we worry about how our crying may affect how others perceive us.[38] Crying in front of others may feel shameful or be suppressed with the worry that our crying may make others feel bad.[39]

People who suppress crying on a regular basis, rather than express their distress by allowing themselves the opportunity to cry, are more likely to suffer burnout in stressful jobs such as nurse or police officer.[40] Research done in several different universities in Germany (Dresden University of Technology, Ulm University, University of Konstanz) on 103 rescue workers showed that suppressed feelings of sadness and ruminations about negative experiences created lasting job stress and stress-related health symptoms. Rescue workers who could feel and accept their distress, on the other hand, showed fewer such symptoms.[41] In these cases, the lack of crying reflects a failure to modulate in the face of interpersonal demands and self-expectations that ultimately dysregulates the emotional experience.[42]

While crying can have parasympathetic releasing and calming effects in modulated and restorative states, people who are depressed and therefore already dysregulated show increased sympathetic and decreased parasympathetic activation when crying. In such cases, dysregulated crying has a pathetic quality that feels to the listener like hopelessness, as if there is nothing that will help and that life is unfulfilling and not worth living.[43] These pathetic forms of crying actually suppress ESA states, as if these cries are used to cover up feeling or redirect them elsewhere. Such cries often occur without tears.

Pathetic, dysregulated cries may seem purposeful, melodramatic, and self-centered. There is no way to really comfort this type of crying, and in fact, you may experience hearing the cry as manipulative. The crier acts needy and hurt in the hope that you will pay attention or yield to a demand. Like crying wolf, these people become tiring after a while, and you may begin to avoid contact with them.

The most distressing type of dysregulated cry for the listener is so-called infantile crying. The person's lips may tremble, and their body tenses up or shakes. It seems like the person is "lost" inside themselves, and we have a feeling of helplessness to reach them. This type of cry may involve not only active suppression of feeling but also dissociative qualities such as leaving the body. There may not be much you can do in this situation except wait for the episode to pass and talk about what happened.

Modulated ESA of Sadness

Modulated forms of crying involve the use of emotional intelligence using TPN thinking. The cries sound more "real" and "authentic," compared to dysregulated "pleas-for-help" cries, in the sense that they are coming from brief moments of parasympathetic letting go into feelings of loss or sadness. As in all modulated felt experience, however, these brief cries are followed by attempts to explain, to understand, to reach out to others verbally for support and sharing.

In situations of modulated sadness, researchers from the Department of Experimental Psychology at the University of Oxford (UK) found that people often explained why they were crying with statements such as "Because I felt that the experience of crying might decrease my distress," "Because I felt that I needed a good cry," "Because I needed support from other people," and "Because I felt that others' reactions would decrease my distress."[44]

Similarly, a sample of cancer patients studied in the Department of Social and Welfare Studies at Linköping University (Norrköping, Sweden) expressed similar explanations for why crying provided them benefits. They described using crying as a way of expressing urgent needs for support or care, or as a release of pent-up emotions when done in a quiet and sorrowful manner.[45]

Modulated crying is indeed helpful under some circumstances. People who express modulated forms of crying are more likely to show improved mood and a sense of relief when they are able to cry and talk about it in front of a trusted person.[46] Crying can elicit help from others and create opportunities for others to be helpful to the person who is crying.[47]

Another study on modulated crying during social and psychotherapeutic situations was done at the Department of Counseling Psychology at the University of Toronto (Canada). The authors conclude that

> *when trauma survivors are able to "stay with" their feelings by expressing them rather than avoiding them, it gives them the opportunity to revise their view of these feelings. With exposure interventions clients do not stay with their painful feelings continuously or indefinitely, but only under controlled circumstances (e.g., during a therapy session) and for periods long enough to have the intensity of their emotional experience and arousal decrease. This enables them to perceive their distress as tolerable and manageable rather than dangerous.[48]*

The conclusion of these studies is that letting ourselves cry with trusted other people can create opportunities for modulated TPN insights in order to "help people to recognize, understand, and interpret their inner subjective states."[49] People can also learn to conceptualize that they were able to cry and that it did not get out of control: that the crying would not go on forever, and that they could develop an increasing ability to tolerate sadness and loss.

Restorative ESA of Sadness

Heaven knows we need never be ashamed of our tears, for they are rain upon the blinding dust of earth, overlying our hard hearts.
—CHARLES DICKENS, *GREAT EXPECTATIONS*, 1860

Restorative crying, again like all forms of restorative felt experience, leads to a transformational state of relief and surrender. According to an interview study of clients and psychotherapists done by a researcher from the Centre for Counselling and Psychotherapy Education in London (UK), restorative crying can lead to a feeling of experiencing something sacred and transformative, compassion and empathy, liberation, free floating and nonfocused awareness, warmth, calm, joy, connection, love, relief, and purification.[50]

The tears from restorative crying have a different physiological composition from tears that bathe the eyes when we blink or get an irritant in the eye, or from other forms of crying. Restorative tears have proteins and stress hormones like the cortisol precursor ACTH. They may, therefore, be a way of flushing out stress-related chemicals and increasing the probability of creating a whole-body relaxation response. Similarly, restorative crying increases parasympathetic and decreases sympathetic activation (the opposite of dysregulated crying) to induce a calming effect.[51]

These effects are most likely to occur when a therapist, or for that matter any person who witnesses crying, behaves in an empathic manner. Being a witness includes not asking people to explain why they are crying, which would lead the person back into modulated ESA. Like all restorative emotions, crying just "is" a feeling and thus beyond thought or explanation.

Silent witnessing of crying is often sufficient to evoke feelings of relief in the crier. Attempts to comfort or soothe the crier tend to suppress the emotion and create dysregulated or modulated feelings and thoughts of shame or doubt about being so open with others. Crying, if it is to have a restorative effect, is fundamentally a way of gaining or regaining a felt connection to one's own experience of sadness, loss, loneliness, and grief.[52]

According to Judith K. Nelson, author of the book *Seeing through Tears: Crying and Attachment,*

> *Crying is above all a relationship behavior, a way to help us get close and not simply a vehicle for emotional expression or release. Crying is not about what we let out but about whom we let in[53] ... In the act of crying, we have love and loss, life and death. Crying holds the opposites: hopelessness and hope, pain and comfort, loneliness and connection.[54]*

A restorative cry is accompanied by deeply felt sensations of warm tears, blurry vision, a sense of vulnerability, and relief in finally just being with our emotions. Restorative cries resonate in sound and feeling within the ESA of both the crier and the listener. Restorative cries have been shown to activate the parasympathetic nervous system, which stimulates tears to flow from the lachrymal glands of the eyes and also stimulates the production of saliva and digestive fluids. Restorative crying tends to reduce heart rate and ease breathing.[55]

The power of restorative grief and crying is illustrated by actor and stand-up comic Marc Maron, who was interviewed in August 2020 about the recent loss of his partner, Lynn Shelton.

> Interviewer: *Do you find it at all difficult to ask for people's sympathies or for acknowledgment of your grief during a global pandemic?*
>
> Marc Maron: *That's one of the reasons I thought it was good to do it. There's nothing but grief around. It's a tough emotion for people to sit in and accept. The one thing the pandemic has given me is time to process and sit with the feelings. I cry every day. The shock and the trauma have dissipated a little bit, so now I deal with the loss. It's been challenging to be in this much sadness in a fairly hopeless world. In terms of really experiencing the feelings that one has with grief and loss, I've had the presence to be in those.[56]*

Imagine that someone close to you has been distressed about something. When you see that person, you offer a hug, and their tears come effortlessly. The person can now feel the pain and grief that had been held back. Then the person's body settles, relaxes, and molds into your arms and body. The person feels relieved, safe, and comforted, flooded with warmth and gratitude, all feelings that you both can share in the present moment. No words are needed.

Shame/Embarrassment

Shame, like pride and guilt, is a so-called self-conscious emotion. While all the other "basic" emotions mentioned previously in this chapter form during the first year of life, self-conscious emotions like shame do not appear until the end of the second year of life, as toddlers become aware of themselves in front of a mirror. At that time, and over the next few years, they begin to notice that if they can see themselves, then other people can see them as well. This is the developmental origin of self-consciousness.

We saw in the previous chapter how children, teens, and young adults are particularly susceptible to feelings of shame about their body's size, shape, and appearance. Older people are not immune from feelings of shame about their self-image, but its intensity and toxicity tend to wane with age, as we grow more comfortable with and become more accepting of ourselves as we are.

Dysregulated ESA of Shame

Shame is an emotion that occurs with the feeling of being observed and exposed in front of others. Dysregulated shame usually occurs with feelings of self-consciousness, self-judgment, and worry or anxiety. When with another person who appears disapproving, we experience shame as toxic and want to deny the feeling and blame or avoid the other person.[57] There is something about the sense that others are seeing us in a negative or judgmental way that promotes anxiety and dysregulation with shame.[58]

The actual felt experience of dysregulated shame includes burning in the cheeks and face, wanting to run or hide, and wanting to cover our face or body. There is often the sense that we are naked from the felt exposure. When we have dreams in which we are naked in groups, it is usually a sign that we have recently had the experience of feeling ashamed.

Another part of the dysregulated shame experience is the feeling that we are alone and abandoned. In these cases, the others who are watching us are not there—at least in our perception of them—to help or support us. The feeling is that we are being seen as objects, less than human. This is the felt experience when people look at our body and not at our face, when we are judged by the color of our skin or by our ethnic or religious identity, or when we are shunned by a group.

Many narratives that have come out of the Black Lives Matter movement in the US and other countries involve the shame of being watched just when walking down the street or going into a market. In these cases, however, the shame is coupled with a sense of menace and fear that goes with a very real history of police and mob violence against Black people. We humans have a long way to go if we are ever to overcome the suspicion, condemnation, imposed restrictions, hatred, and violence against women and ethnic, religious, racial, and gender-identity minorities.

Modulated ESA of Shame

Like all modulated emotional experiences, we can use our TPN to buffer the pain of the situation. We can think of clever things to say to people who are observing us, or we can take steps to avoid an unwanted gaze. This might include dressing in a way that hides the shapes and contours of the body, not working out in a gym with lots of other people around to watch, avoiding mirrors, not walking in places that do not feel safe, or spending most of our time with safe others.

An example of modulating shame experiences comes from research done at the University of British Columbia (Canada). Surveys were collected in a major North American city at three locations—a nightclub, a shopping mall, and on a university campus—from 497 people between the ages of eighteen and twenty-six (209 females, 280 males). This particular group was chosen because they told researchers that they had previously purchased condoms. Sixty-four percent of respondents (70.8 percent of females and 58.9 percent of males) indicated feeling moderate embarrassment when buying condoms, and this percentage declined with age and experience.

These individuals typically found ways to modulate the experience of shame (e.g., "I spend as little time in the aisle as possible," "I go to the shortest cash line," "I steal condoms," "I go to health clinics," "I go to the cashier closest to my age," or "I go with my partner").[59] A similar study done at the Department of Marketing at Old Dominion University (Norfolk, Virginia, USA) showed that people tend to choose cashiers of the same sex and that women are more likely than men to purchase additional products in which to hide or mask the presence of condoms from other customers.[60]

Modulated shame involves the same kinds of felt experiences as dysregulated shame. The difference is that we don't allow ourselves to get destabilized by the feelings. In dysregulated shame, the feelings continue to burn into our awareness long after the burning in our cheeks has subsided. In modulated shame, we are able to limit how much the feelings touch us or get to us.

This works best when, like the condom buyers, we anticipate feeling ashamed and take steps to minimize the impact. We go into the store where we might feel anxious and self-conscious and we get out as quickly as possible, finding the checkout route that is least likely to exacerbate the shame experience. When we get outside the store, we can deliberately take a few breaths to calm ourselves, and we might even feel victorious that we took this risk and succeeded.

Our ability to modulate shame only works when we have the opportunity to escape the situation and find ways to settle and recover. In many of the examples of dysregulated shame, however, there is literally no easy escape route. If we are overweight, a person of color, a gender nonconformist, or handicapped by birth complications or by an accident or trauma, we are always visible and always being observed when outside of our homes and safe spaces.

Restorative ESA of Shame

After reading about dysregulated and modulated shame, and also because shame is inherently a self-conscious emotion, you might wonder if there could be such a thing as restorative shame. In dysregulated and modulated shame, we typically are faced with other people who are, in fact, judging or condemning us with their gaze, thoughts, and intention.

Restorative shame *always and only* occurs when the people who are watching us are compassionate about our embarrassment, caring toward us, or wanting in some way to support or help us. In this sense, restorative shame is the same as restorative crying and sadness: it can elicit support and comfort from other people, which promotes a sense of acceptance and relief.

In South and East Asian cultures, shame is seen as an essential emotion that brings people together. Parents in Taiwan, for example, use their children's experiences of shame as opportunities to teach them about building awareness of others, respecting others' needs, and helping them accept and move past their own interpersonal failings.[61] A therapist from the Department of Psychiatry at Rinsen Clinic (Tokyo, Japan) states that "in the Japanese language 'a person who does not know shame' is equivalent to a 'thick-skinned' and 'insensitive' person who is practically unfit for society."[62]

According to Sana Sheikh of the School of Psychology and Neuroscience at the University of St. Andrews (Fife, UK), who has studied shame in China,

Shame-sharing, in which one's shame extends to others, reflects an interdependent self-construal prevalent in collectivist cultures. Shame in these contexts is likely a painful experience. However, the

extended network of others implicated by one's shame and their dependence on the shamed individual also creates a sense of obligation and responsibility toward those who are shamed. This responsibility motivates restorative behaviors such as self-improvement to bring oneself—and by extension, others—out of the shameful state. The obligation inherent in shame-sharing focuses the person on social relationships and the social context rather than on one's internal attributes, making it easier to effect change and make reparations.[63]

Unfortunately, too many people in Western societies are preoccupied with fostering self-reliance and individualism. With respect to shame, this means that Westerners, compared with Asian peoples, are more likely to feel alone, exposed, or abandoned in dysregulated experiences of shame. Fortunately, however, there are many relationship contexts in Western cultures that share this Asian idea of the restorative nature of shame.

Research done at the University of California, Berkeley (USA), used a large sample of undergraduate students in psychology and sociology courses, coming from a wide range of racial and ethnic groups, in a series of studies exploring the meaning of shame. Most of the students who viewed images of shame in others rated the embarrassed person as being more sociable and approachable compared to images of people displaying different emotions or no emotions at all. Because they viewed the embarrassed images as people who are more socially available, the students said that they would be more willing to offer resources to them and to spend time with them compared to the people in the images that did not express shame.[64]

The results of this research mean that most people in Western cultures are perhaps more accepting of our shame than we think. When we feel ashamed, our first impulse is to hide and protect ourselves. In fact, if we let ourselves look, we might see that our embarrassment makes the person in front of us want to get closer to us. It is exactly this possibility—that shame can bring honesty and closeness into human relationships—from which restorative interpersonal experiences may arise.

As discussed in the previous chapter, children whose parents did not judge or shame them for their food choices or their body image were able to develop healthier eating habits and become less picky eaters. In optimal child-rearing situations, when children feel ashamed at home or have a shameful experience outside the home, parents can meet these feelings with love and compassion to create life-affirming and restorative growth experiences.

Discussions between parents and children, or between romantic partners or friends, about shameful experiences can lead to helpful modulated strategies for managing shame the next time it occurs. Restorative shame, however, can only occur when our parent, partner, or friend can see our tears, our worry, our exposure, and simply embrace us and surround us with love and acceptance. At that point, our self-consciousness can transform into self-love and forgiveness. Sure, discussions are likely to follow, and they help develop those modulated coping strategies, but these strategies are more likely to strengthen us if they arise from a place of shared love and respect.

Summary and Conclusions

You may have noticed while reading this chapter that whether an emotion is experienced as dysregulated, modulated, or restorative often depends on the relational context in which emotional feeling may occur. Dysregulated emotions are more likely to occur when we feel, because of past history and belief or because of actual current circumstances, that the people we are with cannot be trusted or have a dismissive or malicious intent toward us. Restorative emotions are most likely when the people around us are fully present, allowing, and sufficiently generous to give us the space, love, and silent witnessing for our emotion to be felt and expressed.[65]

This is because emotions are fundamentally social experiences. Our expressions signal to others something about our inner state and are meant, ideally, to foster mutually supportive interpersonal bonds of attachment and empathy. When either person is dysregulated, this system can go awry, pushing people away from us or pushing ourselves away from others. Modulated emotions are in a middle ground, sometimes allowing for helpful discussions and mutual understanding and sometimes resulting in separations and detachments.

Experiences of Restorative Embodied Self-Awareness

In Their Own Words

Unlike the previous chapters in which we looked at the differences and shifts between states of dysregulated, modulated, and restorative embodied self-awareness, this final chapter focuses primarily on restorative ESA. While previous chapters provided some examples of individuals' descriptions of their different states of ESA, this chapter contains personal descriptions of what it feels like to be in restorative ESA.

The writings quoted for this chapter do not specifically mention the word *restoration* but were chosen because they illustrate the basic principles of restorative ESA as described in chapter 3: there is a felt parasympathetic state of rest; the feelings come spontaneously and without TPN (task-positive network) or DMN (default-mode network) conceptual thought, focused attention, or planning; and we are able to slow down, let go, surrender to being fully in the moment, to allow our attention to be broad and free-floating, in other words, without "doing," effort, or deliberate control.

The subtitle of this chapter, "In Their Own Words," reflects how—after offering a great deal about the conceptual and research bases of the three states of ESA—this book closes with a series of reports of personal experiences. This is meant to ground the previous chapters in real-life situations of restoration. These personal experiences can also serve as a guide, should you choose to take these words to heart, of how it may feel to you to engage in restorative experiences.

In the end, you are the ultimate judge of where you are on the spectrum of the three states. As discussed earlier, if you are trying to convince yourself that you are in a restorative state, then it is almost certain that you are in a modulated state, where thinking and doing take precedence over letting go and just feeling. Take the words of others included in this chapter inside yourself and see what resonates, what brings you into a deeper connection with yourself, or what moves you to tears.

The Restorative Experience of Being in Nature

As discussed in chapter 3, the restorative experience of awe often comes from being in a natural environment. The natural world has been shown to bring us in touch with ourselves and remind us what is important in our lives. Nature enhances our sense of connection and belonging of the self—a feeling of oneness—between ourselves and other people, animals, plants, trees, and Earth itself. Rabbi Lawrence Kushner, in his book *Honey from the Rock*, writes,

> *The wilderness ... demands being open to the flow of life around you. A place that demands being honest with yourself ... being present with all of yourself.*
>
> *In the wilderness your possessions cannot surround you. Your preconceptions cannot protect you. Your logic cannot promise you the future. Your guilt can no longer place you safely in the past. You are left alone each day with an immediacy that astonishes, chastens and exults. You see the world as if for the first time.*[1]

Talking about her relationship to the earth, and particularly to stones, author Louise Livingstone of Canterbury Christ Church University (UK) writes that

> *something happens to me when I am connected with stones; something is exchanged between myself and them which leaves me with a greater sense of wellbeing and calm. It is as though I am in the presence of some kind of ancient wisdom that comforts and soothes me, and I do feel that I am equally as important in the life of the stone.*[2]

Miriam-Rose Ungunmerr-Baumann is an Aboriginal Australian activist, educator, and founder of the Merrepen Arts Centre in Nauiyu, Northern Territory, Australia. She writes about the Aboriginal quality of relating to others and nature.

> *In our language this quality is called dadirri. It is inner, deep listening and quiet, still awareness. Dadirri recognises the deep spring that is inside us. We call on it and it calls to us. It is something like what you call "contemplation."*
>
> *When I experience dadirri, I am made whole again. I can sit on the river bank or walk through the trees; even if someone close to me has passed away, I can find my peace in this silent awareness. There is no need of words.*
>
> *The contemplative way of dadirri spreads over our whole life. It renews us and brings us peace. It makes us feel whole again. Our Aboriginal culture has taught us to be still and to wait. We do not try to hurry things up. We let them follow their natural course— like the seasons.*[3]

There is something unique about being outside that brings us back to the present moment of feelings and sensations. Outside, it is somehow easier to shed the ruminative thoughts and worries, the inner dialogues and routine mental ruts, and just feel our body in concert with nature. Walking through the desert near the Great Salt Lake in Utah (USA), Alycia Scott Zollinger—a body psychotherapist, somatic movement educator and therapist, and a certified yoga instructor living in Seattle, Washington—describes her restorative experience.

The withheld emotions dating back to my experiences as a child through to the current day surfaced. I collapsed. I felt empowered. I sang out and I cried in despair of the harshness. The heat of the desert both exhausted and warmed me. I continued down to the water. The water was cold. Instead of stepping away, I stepped in. As my expressions processed through me, I dedicated myself to breathe and be within the connection with myself, the water, sand, and rock below me. In what felt like a short time (that also encompassed decades), my breath brought me into an embodied peacefulness. The serenity translated into a somatic buoyancy of beautiful pleasure. Suddenly, I was floating on a branch in cold water, completely ecstatic in awe and gratitude.[4]

A similar connection with nature was experienced by Carol Burstein, a body-centered psychotherapist.

I feel liquid. Familiar boundaries dissolve. I sense an exquisite resonance with fellow breathers in this crucible, crickets and birds outside, palm trees swaying with the gentle breeze. I have also discovered subtle intrinsic movement that seems to reside outside my own emotional circuitry; its sensations are impersonal. As I dwell in the silent, felt world of sensation, I feel an underlying evolutionary connectedness of tissues within and life forms outside of me.[5]

Even simulations of the natural world can have similar calming effects. During the COVID-19 crisis, when health care workers were under an unusual amount of stress, a former triage tent was set up to create simulations of nature and placed just outside the entrance to the emergency department at Mount Sinai Beth Israel hospital in Manhattan (New York City, USA). In this tent, a place

where doctors and nurses once tested patients at sterile medical stations, they now lounge in leather recliners surrounded by plants, watching one of nine landscapes. They just need to say where they want to be, and the voice-activated system transports them to the scene. Dr. Dahlia Rizk [one of the health care personnel who came to the tent] prefers the sun rising over the ocean, because it reminds her of her family home in Florida. Each scene has its own soundscape designed by music therapists, and diffusers fill the space with lavender, chamomile and other scents. "You go from hearing beeps and vents and whistles and all the intensity on the ward, with the bright lights, to this serene space," said Dr. Rizk. "Suddenly something happens that really allows you to decompress almost immediately."

In a survey of about 500 visitors to this triage tent, hospital officials said self-reported stress dropped 60 percent after just fifteen minutes in the tent's rooms. Other forms of self-directed stress relief, such as meditation, generate about a 30 percent drop, and meditation practice requires taking the time to learn how to meditate.[6] So even artificial "natural" environments can have an almost immediate restorative effect of rest, calm, and peace.

Restorative Sexuality

Dysregulated sexuality, and dysregulated social engagement in general, may include using and abusing others, power plays, dominance, harassment, or inflicting harm on self and others. Alternatively, one can feel inadequate, "not enough" or "less than," shame, withdrawal, avoidance, passivity, unwanted submission, or a tuning out of the other person. These feelings can create ways of avoiding sex, not talking about sex or sexual problems, or detachment, dissociation from the body, lack of interest in sex or inability to achieve erection or orgasm, premature ejaculation, pain during intercourse, or nonconsensual sexual aggression.

Modulated sexuality can be mutually playful, challenging, creative, exploratory, edgy—or, on the other hand, tinged with uncertainty, vigilance, self-consciousness, mismatched expectations, power, or submission, perhaps cycling with moments of ease and letting down one's guard. Modulated sexuality is typically mixed in with conversation plus TPN and DMN thoughts about sex, body image, sexual fantasies, or anything else. The sex act may be filled with thoughts, except perhaps during the moment of orgasm, after which the thoughts return leaving no room for peace and rest.

In comparison, restorative sexuality is unselfconscious and honest, and it can be both intense and affectionate. It is always followed by a deep state of contentment, oneness, ease of being together, love, and the awe of being so deeply connected to another person. Restorative sexuality is typically warm, respectful, caring, mutual, and free of pressure to perform or to reach a specific goal. If you are thinking about what to do or say, or trying to make the right moves with your partner, you are more likely engaged in modulated sexuality.

One example of a method to encourage restorative sexuality is called *orgasmic meditation*. This is a practice of having a partner of either gender gently stroke a woman's clitoris for about fifteen minutes with no other goal other than to feel, connect, and be present.[7] Nicole Daedone, in *Slow Sex: The Art and Craft of the Female Orgasm*, explains:

> *In Orgasmic Meditation we learn to shift our focus from thinking to feeling, from a goal orientation to an experience orientation. This shift turns all our expectations about sex on their head, exchanging "faster" and "harder" for "slower" and "more connected."*[8]

Kimerer LaMothe, a dancer and philosopher and author of the book *Why We Dance*,[9] writes about restorative sexuality in terms of what she calls "life-enabling touch" in her previous book, *What a Body Knows: Finding Wisdom in Desire*.

> *If we are touched with care and tenderness, empathy and tact, we may be more likely to remain open to what we feel. We may be more inclined to cultivate our sensory awareness as a guide to health and well-being. We may be more willing to breathe into our emotions with a respect that allows us to discern wisdom in the fiery heart of our desires for food, sex, and spirit, and move with it....*
>
> *Desire. An onrush of sensation flares through us, flooding all registers of awareness. We may think we are drawn in by the shape of a face, the curve of a back, the length of a leg ... We may imagine that our desire is merely for sex or for love. But when that surge blasts through us, such distinctions mean little. The eruption of vitality ... draws us into and out of ourselves ... We find ourselves impelled to take risks, bear secrets, and blurt out crazy ideas. We allow ourselves to be seen by another. We feel joy that unfolds us in generosity.*[10]

A study on sexuality beliefs and experiences was done at the Graduate School of Creative Art Therapies at the University of Haifa (Israel) on a group of nine couples who participated in twelve sessions of dance/movement therapy. Couples talked about the importance of a sense of security, lack of self-consciousness, and "magical" compatibility that makes sex a restorative experience.

> *One participant (in a relationship for 5 years) describes the feeling of delight and letting go, engendered from her security in the total dependence on another: "All the tension is released from my body when I close my eyes, I'm on a high. Closing my eyes and being led is the most freeing/pleasant state. He leads excellently and I also manage to rely on him and to free my body and to laugh all the while." Her partner emphasizes that her feeling of security with him arouses confidence in his body's dependence and relaxation in the encounter with her: "(When I close my eyes) I feel the full weight of your body and your confidence in me to carry you along ... the feeling that you can lean and depend on me."*[11]

Restorative sexuality is perhaps the most effective path to maintaining sexual intimacy in older adults. Body changes in erectile function, vaginal lubrication, and sagging skin can lead in many cases to the dysfunction and disappearance of sexual intimacy in older couples. On the other hand, when couples are willing to listen to their body's changes and desires and listen to each other, sexual pleasure can continue into old age.

Penetration and intercourse may not be possible for some people. For them, mutual genital touching and masturbation, oral sex, petting, fondling, massaging, and the use of sexual literature, photos, or videos can all be part of maintaining desire, reaching orgasm, and sharing longer periods of time in close physical contact without the need to perform or to behave a certain way or to meet some idealistic notion of what sex "should" be.[12]

This is illustrated by the following personal accounts of older women, part of a study done at the Australian Research Centre on Sex, Health and Society at La Trobe University (Melbourne).

> *"I'm quite happy to have what you might call a fuck, I mean it's great and to feel horny and to have somebody else feel attracted and passionate ... But I also probably desire more whole body intimacy. I love to be touched, to be stroked, to be massaged (age 69)."*[13]

> *"We care for each other. We sleep together, and we curl up together. We touch each other, all these things, which is basically what intimacy is (age 78)."*[14]

"There's not a lot of sex anymore and it doesn't really worry me. You know masturbation is still perfectly available (age 61)."[15]

"The women I've known, like in this stage of my life, are not frightened of sex. I reckon it's probably the best time in your life actually (age 57)."[16]

Another, similar study done at the Universities of Canterbury and Auckland (New Zealand) on older men revealed a similar shift with age to more restorative forms of sexuality and intimate connection.

"For many years I guess all it was about was coming … without even really knowing anything about helping your partner to come, but then over time that changed … with the passage of time just the pleasure of being together when you're having sex with somebody, or with masturbating, just masturbating really quite slowly and feeling a sort of tingle spread over one's body [age 68]."[17]

"I suppose it's like a good wine, it improves with age … More relaxed outlook on making love … whereas perhaps years ago it might have been more aggressive and now it can be, you know, more gentle and loving … You think now how silly you were to adopt that attitude [laughs] because … it's a pity that you've taken 40-odd years or something like that to learn that hey, it doesn't have to be rushed to get enjoyment from it … I feel that probably our sex now is some of the best that we've ever experienced … I can't really say it's because of our age, ah, it's because of closeness, perhaps, you know, taking time, not rushing things … It's just been more satisfying [age 66]."[18]

The adaptations that older couples make in creating more satisfying and restorative sexual intimacy are similar when one or both members of the couple are suffering from an illness that may impair or limit sexual activity. This might include forms of mental illness such as bipolar or obsessive-compulsive disorders, Parkinson's and other neuromotor impairments, breast or prostate cancer, injuries that impair sensorimotor function such as erectile dysfunction, or stroke and other neurological impairments of felt experience and movement.[19] Sex therapies, sexual surrogacy, and other related healing practices can assist couples in finding adaptations to their current conditions.

Restoration in Body-Centered Therapies

There are many forms of body-centered therapy and education. This section is not meant to be inclusive of all such forms. Rather, selections were chosen based on what was found in an online literature search. This search was not meant to be comprehensive or representative but rather simply to find a few, hopefully compelling, personal testimonies that reflected in some way what seemed to be an experience of restoration.

In a study of trauma-sensitive yoga done at Tufts University Counseling and Mental Health Service (Medford, Massachusetts, USA), many trauma survivors talked about how the yoga practice helped them be more present in their embodied experiences.

> *"I definitely feel more connected to my body in that I don't run on autopilot all the time. I think it allowed me to be patient in my anger, to sit with it. Practicing yoga definitely has allowed me to— not only with anger, but with a lot of things—given me the ability to sit with things for longer periods of time."*[20]

Body-oriented psychotherapy is a broad field encompassing many different approaches, all of which converge on the use of talking and an emphasis on felt experience and on the body and movement. In a study of six patients with schizophrenia done at the Clinic for General Psychiatry at the University of Heidelberg (Germany), participants reported how the therapy had helped them feel more at home in their own embodiment.

> *Patient 1: "And there one feels the body again much more intensively ... How shall I say ... Otherwise one does not feel the body at all, it is always fully unconscious. Somehow movement brings me body awareness. That I can feel my body and that I can feel it as nicely activated and relaxed."*

> *Patient 2: "I feel safer and more confident in my body. And one has a safer stand, one is more inside oneself. Otherwise one is always in the head or in conversation, and there only thinking is required. And there is the body, and one is more centered; I see it so ... And this is not obvious but rather subtle that one feels centered."*[21]

Barbara Holifield, a Jungian analyst and body psychotherapist from San Francisco (California, USA), writes that her work with

> *the kind of knowing that arises from a full-bodied awareness is like a balm for the soul: clear, direct and immediate ... working with the body in psychotherapy can access sources of healing and creativity which are difficult to reach through verbal means alone.*[22]

Another study from the University of Heidelberg was done at the treatment center for refugees called REFUGIO in Munich, Germany. The center offers a combination of dance/movement therapy and verbal psychotherapy done in both individual and group sessions. One case, described below by the therapist, is about an Albanian woman from Kosovo. In a group counseling session, this woman shared that she had been raped by a Serbian soldier during the Serbian persecution of Albanians in Kosovo during the 1998–1999 war. After she talks about the rape, this trauma survivor (called "the narrator" in the excerpt) and other women begin crying until there is a pause. The therapist guiding the group writes,

> *Using this change I ask the narrator if she wishes to hear from the others. She looks and nods at me. I then ask the women to feel free to share their thoughts and feelings. Immediately, several women begin to speak but then let the oldest woman go first. She expresses her compassion and utters consolations by reminding the narrator of the mercy of God. Some others join her and the neighboring women put their hands on the narrator's arms and say that this is really terrible. Meanwhile, the narrator's crying becomes calmer and she blows her nose, appearing more collected. After some time she raises her gaze, pulls herself up, and looks around. Slowly and increasingly calm, her gaze moves from one woman to the next. She utters her thanks in a calm voice. The others answer with murmurs of empathy. Then, the narrator turns to me with a clear gaze and says that "it was good."*[23]

Aside from illustrating the healing effects of embodied therapies and touch, this example shows the restorative power of simple, wordless acceptance of common suffering during interpersonal interactions. The therapist, narrator, and group members—simply by giving time and space for the narrator to feel herself and the acceptance of others—were all able to find a sense of calm, peace, and safety in the group.

A study of the effects of an embodied (physiotherapeutic) approach to psychiatric rehabilitation was done in the Department of Physiotherapy at Lund University (Sweden). The researchers interviewed forty-four participants who described how feeling their embodied self-awareness was crucial to their recovery. One participant said,

> *"When my awareness is centered in my body, in myself, it gives me a different sense of security and warmth with others. I can accept the changes both within me and outside of me if I can keep this contact with myself. I am now much less afraid of other people and I can see things as they really are even if it hurts."*[24]

Authentic movement is a way of allowing movement to be inspired by felt experience and being witnessed by others in a one-to-one therapeutic setting or in a group as it is happening. Typically, the person's eyes are closed to allow for more open attention to the multiplicity of feelings, sensations, movement impulses, images, memories, and/or sounds that are arising spontaneously. The witness "holds" the mover with presence and a steady gaze while simultaneously attending to their own embodied experience. Tina Stromsted, a Jungian analyst, psychotherapist, dance/movement therapist, and somatic/movement educator and therapist in San Francisco, California (USA), describes one of her experiences in authentic movement in this way:

> *After moving this way for several minutes, I feel a warm glow wash through me. My mouth fills with a sweet taste and I hear a kind of buzz within me that reminds me of the sound that bees make around a hive. It's as though they are circulating throughout my body in my bloodstream ... or is it my nervous system ... or perhaps my energetic body? Though the specific "location" is unclear, what is undeniable is how full and peaceful, yet vibrantly alive I feel ... With this resonating awareness, I begin to weep—sweet tears of gratitude, which give me a felt connection to myself, to everyone in the room and, simultaneously, to all of life.*[25]

Here Stromsted shares the experience of one of her students who was engaged in authentic movement practice in a group setting. While contained

by supportive, nonjudgmental witnesses, "Keith" was able to access his embodied experience in ways that had previously been too frightening for him to
feel or to bring to consciousness. Keith reports:

> *On my knees, anger rises up in me. I get up and begin to walk
> across the room and then pace back and forth. I feel very agitated
> and want to explode and let whatever is holding me so tight come
> pouring out. Then something happens so naturally that I am not
> even aware of the change. The anger and agitation give way to a
> sadness that feels as far away as it is present. I sit down and lean
> against the wall, feeling small and innocent, and begin rubbing my
> right leg. I am lost in this moment for a few minutes when all at
> once I realize what I am doing. Tears come to my eyes.*[26]

Emotion regulation psychotherapy helps people feel their embodied
experiences of dysregulated anxiety while gradually creating opportunities
to find and feel the "true" emotions that trigger the anxiety. The goal is to be
able to help the client self-regulate in the face of uncomfortable or traumatic
felt experiences.[27]

> *"It's like more integration of a releasing of that thought as well as
> 'okay, am I thinking? Is it my emotions? Is it pain?' But how about
> just like existing in that feeling? ... Here you're still judging and
> thinking ... and doing ... rather than just: it's there."*

> *"I've just been less judgmental of myself, being more aware of my
> thoughts and what I attach, what I think and assign to everything.
> So, I've seen a decrease in my judgment and analyzing of situa-
> tions and just sort of letting them be. And that's definitely helped
> me: it decreases my stress, it helps me be more open to different
> possibilities."*[28]

An interview study of clients who had received emotion-focused therapy was done at the Department of Clinical Psychology at the University
of Bergen (Norway). Emotion-focused therapy is a form of humanistic psychotherapy that uses interpersonal empathy between client and therapist to
help clients transform dysregulated emotions into modulated or restorative
emotions. This study—much like the earlier example of group therapy for

refugees from Kosovo—shows that interpersonal trust and a felt sense of safety with the therapist were crucial ingredients in finding restoration.

> *"I was listened to. I felt that when I cried, she [the therapist] almost sat there and cried together with me. I felt there was a strong connection, which made it easy for me to open up. Even though I was prepared to talk about my problems, still, it became even easier. Safety to open up, and there was something about how the therapist acted. I feel I have been receiving a lot from her. She was there for me. It has been very close and nice, and very supportive. Very safe."[29]*

And a similar process can occur in couples therapy when people who have not been able to share and support each other emotionally begin to open up to each other. Francine Lapides, a psychotherapist from Felton, California (USA), reports on one case as follows:

> *He begins to sob, "I can't take this anymore. I'm not a person, my needs don't get addressed." "Notice what's happening," I suggest, "your voice, your body and where and how you feel this pain. And try to look at Eleanor, try to hold her gaze." I sense it's safe to do this because she appears, as I glance at her, to have managed to hear the accusation without losing her focus on his pain. She leans in again, coming close to his face until he looks up and then she smiles reassuringly, and mirrors his sad expression. For the first time in over 2 months of therapy, they have a tender moment here in front of me. She gathers him in, and he cries and then he apologizes and thanks her for something I cannot quite hear. "You just thanked her Leonard?" I inquire. "Yes," he says, "for letting me be the one who falls apart."[30]*

Similar feelings of relief and forgiveness can occur when being reunited with a loved one after an absence (like a business trip, vacation, or hospitalization) or a repair after a breakup. The tears of joy and relief are mixed with the memory of the grief of having been alone or left behind or feelings of abandonment.

Another variation on embodied approaches to therapy is called *mindful awareness in body-oriented therapy*. In a study at the School of Nursing at the University of Washington (Seattle, USA), therapists described clients' experiences during sessions. In one case,

> *the therapist asks what else she [the client] is noticing. The client, after a long pause responds, saying, "I feel very peaceful." The client then adds that it's been a long time since she's felt so calm inside. The therapist asks her to notice the entire state of her internal body in this experience of calm and peace. The client responds by saying she feels a sense of continuity from her head to her feet; a sense of being whole. She continues noticing her interoceptive experience and says, in a surprised voice, "I have no worries, it is as though my entire being is calm."[31]*

Some forms of body-centered treatment involve both touch and talk. In a study of a technique called *mindful body awareness*, also done at the School of Nursing at the University of Washington, clients described their restorative experience during sessions in the following way:

> *"Unbelievable, when [the therapist] had her hand on my heart and shoulder and I was breathing and becoming aware of my heart/heartbeat, I felt the most incredible sensation of levitation—rising into light. I felt happy and almost like I was going to heaven—no exaggeration."[32]*

> *"I could 'feel' more acutely the sensations that are able to be felt. I was able to feel again that feeling of lightness, of levitating, being carried into the air and into a light of some sort. It was calm and beautiful. The tears I felt welling up—in gratitude toward a connection with my spiritual side."[33]*

Another embodied modality that is sometimes used in nursing practice is called *caring touch*. This is a gentle massage intended to stimulate interoceptive touch receptors in the the skin and muscles without applying direct pressure to or stretching muscles. In a study on caring touch done at the short-term emergency ward at Karolinska University Hospital (Huddinge, Sweden), interviews were done with forty-one patients who had experienced a motor vehicle accident with minor injuries.

> *During a trauma, patients experienced their body and soul as being "scattered." Patients became aware of this disconnect between body*

and mind during the Caring Touch treatments: "And then the treatment put together all the scattered pieces of my puzzle back," and gave them a feeling of wholeness: "It gives a feeling of coming together ... the soul gets back into the body again."

"This massage is about the soul, after the accident the soul is damaged, the body is here ... it is about your soul and your mind, and massage helps that part, of course helps against pain, but most of all it's the part touching your soul, you relax, you forget, you become as you once were."[34]

Rosen Method bodywork is another form of therapy that uses both touch and talk with the goal of enhancing the clients' embodied self-awareness. In chapter 4 (p. 144), there was a report of previously unpublished data on a study I had done on five clients with low-back pain who were given sixteen sessions of Rosen Method bodywork. Client experiences of modulation and restoration were revealed during post-treatment interviews cited in chapter 4.

Following are some previously published observations by the practitioners who worked with these clients, based on notes written by the practitioners after each of the sixteen sessions. These quotes are chosen because they seemed to reflect the practitioners' observations of states of restorative ESA in these clients.

She told me about the one thing that had inspired her last week. From there, everything in her body shifted. More breath, softening of the muscles in her neck. I asked her to notice the experience she was having in her body so that she would know (could learn to recognize) that this is a path for her. She said she makes everything negative, but here, in her body was the breath and the inspiration that had been missing.

Her body is very responsive and her thought(s)/mind is slowly, very slowly, beginning to listen. She was able then to stay longer in the heart-felt sensations. At the end of the session she said the new awareness was like a baby that needed nurturing.

The hopelessness, the failure are so deep and authentic. I can feel the up-welling pretty far inside her. I wait while she feels and then say back, "Everything you did, nothing worked, you felt hopeless." She and I connected, her chest drops slightly, being witnessed

comes through for her and for me. Here at the end is the real jewel:
hopeless, impotent about someone she really, really loves and who
really loved her.[35]

This last example shows that restorative ESA is not always about feeling good. It is about simply feeling whatever we feel in the present moment without any intervening thoughts or interpretations, feelings that bring a sense of relief.

Next are some quotes from other research studies in which Rosen Method bodywork clients were interviewed about their experiences. Each client interviewed had received at least twenty treatment sessions from the same practitioner, although each of the clients had a different practitioner.

"I feel like in that moment, it's not just this connection between me
and B. [her practitioner], but it's this connection between me, and
the practitioner, and this greater source and being. Most times, it's
that peaceful feeling of that connection. It's very meditative."[36]

"I realized that I could think about what I felt in talk therapy, but
it was an intellectual process. Now with Rosen Method therapy, I
have learned to discern what I think I feel and what I really can
feel. I didn't even know that I can actually feel myself until now. I
only knew what I could think. Now I can feel myself, feel love for
myself, know that I am present, that I do exist, in a visceral way.
I would say it takes my breath away, but truth is, it gives me …
breath … the safety to breathe more fully, more deeply. And all
the sensations are … in color now, so to speak, as if they had been
black and white before."[37]

"In the session, no matter what's been going on, how anxious I've
been feeling, how upset I am about something, I can just kind of
let go within … I can feel myself starting to relax and I just feel so
supported and so safe. It's hard to even describe adequately … I
find myself wanting to just stay like that like forever. (Laughs) …
in that place where I don't have to do anything else. Just relax and
just breathe. And feel."[38]

"This work has helped me really feel things viscerally and integrate
things so they're not just like this concept like, 'Oh, of course, I

know that.' No. To actually feel, to experience it in my body. Then, the whole world is different.... And it doesn't ever go back. You're changed forever!"[39]

"There's kind of a deeper, quiet, knowing that there are places in me that I'm not even aware of ... And it's almost like they are pathways into the spirit, or a pathway into a very deep, hidden self."[40]

These quotes speak to links between restorative ESA and the transformative power of awe, grace, something bigger than the self and the other, safety, peace, surrender, breath, depth, and quiet. And one client's report echoes a point that has been made in earlier chapters of this book: that sustained restorative ESA can be the entry point for a permanent and lasting change in one's state of being: "the whole world is different.... And it doesn't ever go back."

Restorative Forms of Meditation

There are many ways of paying attention to the body that fall under the very broad heading of *meditation*. There are countless ancient practices and philosophies of meditation. Virtually every country in East and South Asia has a unique legacy of multiple traditions, just as most countries in Africa and in North and South America have indigenous practices related to connecting with self and with the earth. In addition, there are many types of Western contemporary meditation practices—most of them based in some way on the ancient traditions—that are becoming increasingly used in conventional and alternative forms of health care.

There is a broad range of resources about these differing traditions and practices. The common designation for many of the Western practices is *mindfulness*, the ability to stay focused on one's feelings and sensations, whether positive or negative, in a nonreactive and nonevaluative manner. As researcher Antonie Lutz and colleagues put it, "Mindfulness meditation practices can be conceptualized as a set of attention-based, regulatory and self-inquiry training regimes cultivated for various ends, including well-being and psychological health."[41]

Most mindfulness practices, in the language of this book, use focused attention that is supported by sympathetic arousal. When this form of attentional focus and training occurs in states of modulated ESA, it can lead to extremely helpful improvements in well-being, emotional intelligence, and self-modulatory strategies for reducing stress and facilitating healing from medical treatments.[42]

On the other hand, mindfulness practice can sometimes slip into dysregulated ESA when attentional focus gets pulled into past trauma, worry, rumination, and pain. David Treleaven, a specialist in the use of meditation for healing trauma, has suggested that "sustained attention to the body can lead to a dissociative, or freeze, response" that he has named "contemplative dissociation."[43] The result is that, without guidance, one can get stuck in the pain and can't get out, leading to prolongation of states of dysregulated ESA.

Anna Lutkajtis at the University of Sydney (Australia) suggests that these potentially harmful effects of meditation have been underreported and that the literature has a strong bias toward mindfulness as universally beneficial. She writes that the adverse effects of mindfulness that have been reported in the scientific literature include "dissociative symptoms; psychosis-like experiences; out-of-body experiences; depersonalization and derealisation; confusion and disorientation; increases in perceived stress and depression; increased false memory susceptibility; links to criminogenic thinking; and exacerbation of traumatic distress."[44]

Most of the research on mindfulness, then, has been about either dysregulation or modulation, using the language of this book. Recall from chapter 1 that meditations using a broad or open way of paying attention to ourselves—when we allow our attention to be called to any form of felt experience that arises—prove to be the most helpful in promoting restorative states.

Vipassana meditation, to take one such example, involves an open and flexible awareness. One usually begins by noticing the physical sensations related to breathing in the abdomen area. From there, as in the exercise in chapter 1 (p. 12), one's attention is allowed to drift to any form of embodied self-awareness that may arise. An interview study was done at the Human Sciences Research Centre at the University of Derby (UK) on people who had at least five years or more of regular practice of vipassana meditation.

"That was my first retreat. And I felt like coming home ... I knew, directly, I knew with all my, with all I am, that this was it."[45]

"So, equanimity for me is that you stay more neutral, you can go back easier; you just acknowledge 'Ok, if it's, whatever is there, the anger, the fear, the joy', so there is less, less and less reaction."[46]

"And this wanting and not wanting creates unrest, creates anxiety ... And all this anxiety and unrest, that slowly diminishes. And then in this calm ... you go even deeper, you find more of this friction, you find more unrest. You also bring that to calm and then go on and on and on and on and on. And, you can go even deeper by going into this ever-changing nature of everything that happens."[47]

A study was done at the School of Psychology, National University of Ireland (Galway) on the experience of forty-one people who had practiced a variety of different forms of meditation or yoga for at least five years. Many of the participants described their growing ability to access restorative states:

It was also noted that "a feeling of love" and "feelings of inner peace and stillness" reciprocally enhance one another—"they are just interconnected, each one enhances the other; one doesn't come first and one doesn't come second—they are sort of together really."[48]

"A sense of deep acceptance" in turn is argued to lead to "a sense of lightness": "once something is accepted then it's released and there's no tension there anymore. So, it's like letting go—there's a lightness in that," which enhances "feelings of peace and calm" through relaxing of conflict.[49]

"It's like letting down the guard—when that comes down—then I'm more available for being kind and compassionate" and more embracing of what people are like: "I think you are embracing all of the world and people that are in it—as they are, warts and all—even if you don't like them and then you treat them kindly and with compassion."[50]

Philip Shepherd, who leads workshops on embodiment and meditation practices, writes in his book *Radical Wholeness: The Embodied Present and the Ordinary Grace of Being,*

The quality of presence cannot be achieved—you discover your presence as you surrender to the Present. And in that surrender you feel its energy shifting in utter ease around you and through you. The Present is underpinned by love; it plays with unfettered spontaneity;

its currents course with ineffable grace; the Present moves with the
joy of being; it is liberated into the expression of truth.[51]

Note that Shepherd's description of the present moment is not something
that we focus on in a deliberate manner. Rather, it is something we surrender
into as we let go of trying, focusing, and doing.

Brother David Steindl-Rast expresses a similar sentiment in his book *The*
Way of Silence: Engaging the Sacred in Everyday Life.

> *Like most of us, most of the time I would have to say that I am not*
> *really present where I am. Instead, I'm 49 percent ahead of myself,*
> *just stretching out to what's going to come, and 49 percent behind*
> *myself, hanging on to what has already passed. There's hardly any*
> *of me left to be really present. Then something comes along that's*
> *practically nothing, that little sandpiper or the rain on the roof,*
> *that sweeps me off my feet and for one split second I'm really pres-*
> *ent where I am. I'm carried away and I'm present where I am. I lost*
> *myself and I found myself, truly myself.*[52]

Again this quote reminds us that states of restorative ESA can only come
about by letting go of the past and future and letting ourselves be called to a
moment of peace, simplicity, and grace. It's not that the rain on the roof is something that takes effortful attention. Rather, it catches us by surprise and becomes
restorative if we open up to experiencing it as a gift, as a sense of wonder or
awe, as the feeling of being swept away to an entirely different reality.

Spirituality

People, like Brother David in the previous paragraphs, who write about what
is named in this book as restorative ESA may refer to their experience as
"spiritual." It's not clear that there is a difference except in the challenge
of describing these states in narrative language. One could say that practicing restorative ESA on a regular basis is a spiritual quest, or that practicing restorative ESA leads to greater awareness of things deemed spiritual:
feelings of connection, compassion, love, gratitude, forgiveness, surrender,
and acceptance. One could also say that spiritual experiences are felt as

fundamentally life changing in ways that bring peace, acceptance, forgiveness, or a sense of oneness: that is, experiences that are restorative.

An increasing number of research studies on health and well-being are taking spiritual and religious practices into account, particularly with regard to the role of these practices in recovery from stress and trauma. People who survive war, genocide, fires, and sinking ships, for example, often mention religion or spirituality as the most important factor in helping them endure. Veterans Affairs medical centers in the United States have found that incorporating religious rituals into treatment facilitates therapeutic outcomes for PTSD and other illness conditions.[53]

Other research shows that the direct participation of the body in religious ritual and practice helps individuals remember and finally feel suppressed emotions from loss and trauma, which enhances embodied self-awareness, which in turn promotes healing of physical and emotional wounds.[54] In the process of recovery, we come to realize that the events surrounding the trauma and the body's protective response to the threat of those events were beyond our control.

The "I" of our conceptual (TPN and DMN) self-awareness—who we think we are, what we think we can do—has to be revised to more accurately reflect what we actually did and felt and lost in that fateful assault by a chunk of the universe much bigger than that "I." Recovery and restoration occur at the point when the "I"—directly and profoundly—feels, accepts, and forgives our human frailties. This is a spiritual and restorative experience, the heart of self-compassion.

Summary and Conclusions

The personal accounts given in this chapter are, by necessity of the process of speaking and writing, in the form of narrative language. As discussed earlier in this book, restorative ESA is beyond the ability of words to describe. It is not logical, and the only thought or language that can come close to it is evocative. This means that the narratives found in this chapter may "reach" some deeper felt experience inside of you, may "touch" you in a way that an emotion arises or you encounter a sense of "truth."

These narratives, therefore, are not meant to explain or to convince you but rather to "find" you.

If you are *thinking* about these examples using TPN modulated thought, if you are wondering if they are or are not instances of a state of restorative ESA, then you are convincing yourself, and maybe even wanting to believe, that this thing called restoration exists. These thoughts come with effort and sympathetic arousal no matter how well modulated they may be. If you are *thinking* "I understand restoration now," then you are not feeling restored in a way that leads to getting the health benefits of parasympathetic ease.

We have the possibility to fully be healed and soothed by our own restorative ESA only when we are completely honest with ourselves about when we are, or are not, genuinely in that restorative state of peace and grace. Only you can discern whether something in this chapter touched you in a more profound way, in a way that took you out of your ordinary modulated self like Brother David's sandpiper.

This may sound easy but it is not. Human thought is astoundingly ubiquitous. Thinking infuses most conscious moments of our lives. It is so pervasive that we can easily become habituated to it, meaning that—like ordinary noise in the environment in which we live—we become so used to it that we can tune it out.

When we pay attention, however, these background thoughts can be "heard" more clearly, and then we have the possibility to discover a pathway toward a more restorative way of being. Again, using Brother David's eloquent language, 49 plus 49 percent of our lives are wrapped up in thinking, planning, remembering, worrying, explaining, and doing. There isn't much space left for surrender, for letting go of this huge weight of our narratively constructed lives.

But what seems like such a tiny space from the viewpoint of modulated ESA is, in fact, infinite when we arrive in restorative ESA. You can allow someone to lead you to the brink, you can be convinced that it is possible to find this vastness of peace, but only you—only you—can feel safe enough to let go. That is the only way to find the hidden treasure of restoration.

I once went to a climbing park with one of my sons and two grandsons. It was built into a dense forest at the edge of Berlin, Germany, where they live.

The trees were studded with ladders, platforms, zip lines, and chutes. We got fitted with harnesses, clamps, hooks, ropes, and gloves. Unlike my accompanying family members, I had not done this before, so they kindly suggested that we choose one of the green courses: the easiest, beginner-level course.

As we were ascending ladders to ever-higher platforms, I noticed that park employees were bringing an older man down in a sling seat using ropes and pulleys. I was also an older man, sixty-eight at the time, I think, so I asked my son about this. "He couldn't do it, I suppose," was his reply. I didn't think much about this since I have been an athlete all my life. As an expert skier, I have no sense of fear pointing my skis directly downhill on the steepest of slopes.

I was enjoying the climb up. We reached the first jumping platform—about forty feet above the ground—where we had to attach our hooks and harness to a zip line and sail about one hundred feet across to another platform on a different tree. My son and grandsons attached, jumped, and were gone. I hooked in, got to the edge of the platform, looked down, and froze.

I was terrified at the height and the prospect of leaping into the void. My skis are always connected to the snow and to the mountain. This was completely different, being so high off the ground. I remembered the other older man, and now I got what must have happened to him, not by a thought but via a very visceral felt experience of dysregulated nausea and paralysis.

Meanwhile, my son was calling out to me from the platform on the other side of the line. "Come on, Dad, you can do it!" My heart was racing, I took a deep breath, and I jumped. Suddenly, there was nothing but exhilaration, expansion, vastness, floating. When I landed, I got lots of hugs and pats on the back, bringing me into a state of restoration from an intense modulated state of flow. The four of us went on to complete the entire course with more zip lines, hanging rope bridges, and ever more ladders and landings. I felt empowered, and we experienced a lot of shared enjoyment.

As I finish this book, I am turning seventy-five. Skiing down the mountains in winter as I have gotten older, I stop more frequently, sometimes going into the woods along the side of a ski run where I come to a full stop, find silence, peace, and restoration as my breath catches up with me and I settle into the wonder of the mountain's power and beauty. Age gives me the freedom—and the need—to rest more often and to be filled up in this way. It's like slower sex and slower eating. Maybe I could not have written this book earlier in my life because I had been too busy, too intense, to let in the immensity of restorative experiences.

Yet, even now, I have never gotten to a point where I can stay in restorative ESA entirely on my own. I need my resources—being with my life partner, my family, friends, and my cat, receiving ESA therapy from a trusted practitioner, getting massage and acupuncture, connecting with clients and students, doing regular exercise and athletics, gardening, appropriate nutrition, medical care, creative work like this writing project and making music, for example—in order to live most fully in each moment: to be engaged and activated in a modulated state and then allow myself to fall into restoration.

Restorative ESA states are temporary: they are like a flower that blooms only for a short time and only if the plant receives the appropriate stimulation of nutrition, water, and sunlight. Restorative ESA states need patience, care, regular practice, and yes, maybe a perspective of life wisdom. They can't be planned or built into a schedule. They just arise, take us, run their course, and fade like petals dropping away.

I give these examples not to suggest that other people should do the same things as I do for support but rather to affirm that each of us has our own issues and vulnerabilities and each of us has to discover what works best for ourselves in our own lives. The important message is that finding and staying present with *our own felt experience in each of the three states of ESA is essential to cultivate our sense of aliveness and health, and that each of us requires support and regular practices to remain embodied, stay empowered, and be restored.*

Maybe it will help you to make some lists?

- Name some of the places/activities that feel most restorative for you (being in nature, meditation, yoga, dance, authentic and other embodied movement practices, sports and exercise, prayer and spiritual practices, music, art, gardening, cooking, eating healthy foods, shopping, being with family and friends, intimate partnerships, etc.), in which you are more able to fully experience your own restorative ESA. Note that these may be different at different times in your life.

- How can you discern whether any of these or other activities is actually guiding you to a state of restorative ESA rather than to a state of modulated or dysregulated ESA? During and after engaging in the activity, do you feel more alive, healthier, relaxed, happy, or more fully yourself; or do you feel tired, drained, stressed, overwhelmed, tense, or sympathetically "up" or "on"? What would you need to feel in your body for an activity to be genuinely restorative?

- Name some of the places/activities that feel more stressful or overwhelming to you. What happens to you in these different places? Can you self-modulate or do you become dysregulated? How can you discern if you are self-modulating or only thinking that you can handle the situation? Can you sense why these things affect you in these specific ways? How might this response be related to previous events in your life? What can you do to minimize these stressors?

- Make a list of possible changes you might make in your life to maximize time for restorative ESA when you feel stressed or overwhelmed. How can you be with other people in ways that help you find restoration (asking for help, asking someone to just listen, saying no, setting boundaries, asking for the kind of touch you need, etc.)? What does it mean for you to make life-affirming choices? What keeps you from making such choices?

Acknowledgments

I am most grateful to the Rosen Method clients and professionals with whom I have worked over the past twenty years. The theme of this book came out of my observations of changing states of embodied self-awareness during Rosen Method bodywork sessions and trainings that I have given. The detailed characteristics and the choice of names of the three states evolved out of my own work and research, and in discussions with my colleague Amanda Blake, my wife Jacqueline Fogel, and my son Menasheh Fogel. I am also thankful for Amanda Blake (Embodied Coaching) and Maud Guettler (Rosen Method bodywork and Somatic Experiencing), who invited me to coteach workshops and webinars with them as I was developing my ideas about these three states of ESA.

I thank the editors of the *Rosen Method International Journal* and the *International Body Psychotherapy Journal* for publishing the first accounts of the three-state model, based on research I have done with Rosen Method bodywork practitioners and clients. I'm also grateful to Manfred Thielen and the organizers of European Congress of Body Psychotherapy for inviting me to present a keynote lecture and a workshop on these three states at their conference in Berlin, Germany, in 2019; to Laurens van Aarle of Coaches Rising for the invitation to present two webinars on this topic for coach training in neuroscience and embodiment in 2019 and 2020; to Maud Guettler and the executive team of the Rosen Institute for inviting me to present two webinars on these three states for Rosen practitioners; and to Mark Walsh and his international team for inviting me to present a webinar on the three states at their Embodiment Conference in October 2020.

I am grateful to Shayna Keyles, my editor at North Atlantic Books, for seeing the promise in my original book proposal and for her wisdom and guidance in transforming that rather incomplete document into this book. As someone who has a lot of experience working with editors and being an editor, it was a gift to find someone like Shayna who understood this project and helped me find the best way to bring it to life. Many thanks also to Trisha Peck, production editor, and Matthew Hoover, copy editor, for listening to my perspective and for their invaluable contributions to bringing this work to completion. Thanks also to Guy Ruggiero for the illustrations and Angela Newman for assistance with the endnote references.

Finally, during this 2020 year of writing, I received a lot of personal support, encouragement, generosity, and love from my life partner, Jacqueline Fogel, and my sons, Dan and Menasheh Fogel, and their partners, Emily Coley and Julia Schlittgen Fogel. I am also indebted to the support and guidance I received from my gifted health care providers—Karen Anderson, Sarah McCormick, Susan Pohl, and Jill Zablocki—for helping me out of my own dysregulated states and through the challenges of balancing the writing process with the effects of living in a pandemic and sociopolitically divided world, and with other life tasks and commitments.

Notes

Chapter 1

1 Alan Fogel, *Body Sense: The Science and Practice of Embodied Self-Awareness* (New York: W. W. Norton, 2013); Philip Shepherd, *Radical Wholeness: The Embodied Present and the Ordinary Grace of Being* (Berkeley, CA: North Atlantic Books, 2017); Mark Walsh, *Embodiment: Moving Beyond Mindfulness* (United Kingdom: Unicorn Slayer Press, 2020).

2 Frank Röhricht et al., "Embodied Cognition and Body Psychotherapy: The Construction of New Therapeutic Environments," *Sensoria* 10, no. 1 (2014): 11–20, https://doi.org/10.7790/sa.v10i1.389.

3 Carolyn Knapp, *Appetites: Why Women Want* (New York: Counterpoint, 2003), 96. See also Emily Payton, "Bodies under Siege: Women, Eating Disorders, and Self-Injurious Behavior" (senior project, Bard College, 2012), https://digitalcommons.bard.edu/senproj_s2012/364/.

4 Yulia E. Chentsova-Dutton and Vivian Dzokoto, "Listen to Your Heart: The Cultural Shaping of Interoceptive Awareness and Accuracy," *Emotion* 14, no. 4 (2014): 666–78, https://doi.org/10.1037/a0036193; Christine Ma-Kellams, "Cross-Cultural Differences in Somatic Awareness and Interoceptive Accuracy: A Review of the Literature and Directions for Future Research," *Frontiers in Psychology* 5 (2014): 1379, https://doi.org/10.3389/fpsyg.2014.01379.

5 Donald Bakal, *Minding the Body: Clinical Uses of Somatic Awareness* (New York: Guilford, 2001).

6 Elaine A. Leventhal et al., "Active Coping Reduces Reports of Pain from Childbirth," *Journal of Consulting and Clinical Psychology* 57, no. 3 (1989): 365–71, http://www.ncbi.nlm.nih.gov/pubmed/2738209.

7 Fogel, *Body Sense*.

8 James D. Laird, *Feelings: The Perception of Self* (New York: Oxford University Press, 2007).

9 Charlotte Selver, "On Being in Touch with Oneself," *United States Association for Body Psychotherapy Journal* 4, no. 1 (2005): 7–9, https://www.ibpj.org/issues/archive/Vol3No1%20USABP%20Journal%202004.pdf.

10 Jian Xu et al., "Nondirective Meditation Activates Default Mode Network and Areas Associated with Memory Retrieval and Emotional Processing," *Frontiers in Human Neuroscience* 8 (2014): 86, https://doi.org/10.3389 /fnhum.2014.00086; Les Fehmi and Jim Robbins, *The Open-Focus Brain: Harnessing the Power of Attention to Heal Mind and Body* (Boston: Trumpeter Books, 2007).

11 Hamid Reza Naghavi and Lars Nyberg, "Common Fronto-parietal Activity in Attention, Memory, and Consciousness: Shared Demands on Integration?," *Consciousness and Cognition* 14, no. 2 (2005): 390–425, https://doi.org /10.1016/j.concog.2004.10.003.

12 Laura E. Berk, "Development of Private Speech among Preschool Children," *Early Child Development and Care* 24, no. 1–2 (1986): 113–36, https://doi.org/10.1080/0300443860240107; David Furrow, "Social and Private Speech at Two Years," *Child Development* 55, no. 2 (1984): 355–62, https://doi.org/10.2307/1129948.

13 Jay A. Seitz, "The Bodily Basis of Thought," *New Ideas in Psychology* 18, no. 1 (2000): 23–40, https://doi.org/10.1016/S0732-118X(99)00035-5, p. 23. See also Lawrence W. Barsalou, "Grounded Cognition," *Annual Review in Psychology* 59 (2008): 617–45, https://doi.org/10.1146/annurev.psych .59.103006.093639.

14 R. Nathan Spreng and Jessica R. Andrews-Hanna, "The Default Network and Social Cognition," in *Brain Mapping: An Encyclopedic Reference, Vol. 3*, ed. Arthur W. Toga (Cambridge, MA: Academic Press, 2015), 165–69, https:// doi.org/10.1016/B978-0-12-397025-1.00173-1.

15 Manos Tsakiris, Gita Prabhu, and Patrick Haggard, "Having a Body versus Moving Your Body: How Agency Structures Body-Ownership," *Consciousness and Cognition* 15, no. 2 (2006): 423–32, https://doi.org/10.1016 /j.neuropsychologia.2010.05.021.

16 Mareike Clos, Nico Bunzeck, and Tobias Sommer, "Dopamine Enhances Item Novelty Detection via Hippocampal and Associative Recall via Left Lateral Prefrontal Cortex Mechanisms," *Journal of Neuroscience* (August 12, 2019): 0495-19, https://doi.org/10.1523/JNEUROSCI.0495-19.2019; Victoria M. Puig and Allan T. Gulledge, "Serotonin and Prefrontal Cortex Function: Neurons, Networks, and Circuits," *Molecular Neurobiology* 44, no. 3 (2011): 449–64, https://doi.org/10.1007/s12035-011-8214-0.

17 Richard Eleftherios Boyatzis, Kylie Rochford, and Anthony Ian Jack, "Antagonistic Neural Networks Underlying Differentiated Leadership Roles," *Frontiers in Human Neuroscience* 8 (2014): 114, https://doi.org/10.3389 /fnhum.2014.00114; Istvan Molnar-Szakacs and Lucina Q. Uddin, "Self-Processing and the Default Mode Network: Interactions with the Mirror Neuron System," *Frontiers in Human Neuroscience* 7 (2013): 571, https:// doi.org/10.3389/fnhum.2013.00571; Judson Brewer, Kathleen Garrison,

and Susan Whitfield-Gabrieli, "What about the 'Self' Is Processed in the Posterior Cingulate Cortex?," *Frontiers in Human Neuroscience* 7 (2013): 647, https://doi.org/10.3389/fnhum.2013.00647.

18 Ines Blix and Tim Brennen, "Intentional Forgetting of Emotional Words after Trauma: A Study with Victims of Sexual Assault," *Frontiers in Psychology* 2 (2011): 235, https://doi.org/10.3389/fpsyg.2011.00235.

19 Boyatzis, "Antagonistic Neural Networks," 114; Michael D. Fox et al., "The Human Brain Is Intrinsically Organized into Dynamic, Anticorrelated Functional Networks," *Proceedings of the National Academy of Sciences* 102, no. 27 (2005): 9673–78, https://doi.org/10.1073/pnas.0504136102; Lucina Q. Uddin et al., "Functional Connectivity of Default Mode Network Components: Correlation, Anticorrelation, and Causality," *Human Brain Mapping* 30, no. 2 (2009): 625–37, https://doi.org/10.1002/hbm.20531.

20 Joseph Campbell, *The Power of Myth* (New York: Anchor Books, 1988), 4.

21 Stuart Shanker, *Reframed: Self-Reg for a Just Society* (Toronto: University of Toronto Press, 2020).

22 Dustin E. Sarver et al., "Hyperactivity in Attention-Deficit/Hyperactivity Disorder (ADHD): Impairing Deficit or Compensatory Behavior?," *Journal of Abnormal Child Psychology* 43, no. 7 (2015): 1219–32, https://doi.org/10.1007/s10802-015-0011-1.

23 Yovanka B. Lobo and Adam Winsler, "The Effects of a Creative Dance and Movement Program on the Social Competence of Head Start Preschoolers," *Social Development* 15, no. 3 (2006): 501–19, https://doi.org/10.1111/j.1467-9507.2006.00353.x.

24 Dawn Podulka Coe et al., "Effect of Physical Education and Activity Levels on Academic Achievement in Children," *Medicine and Science in Sports and Exercise* 38, no. 8 (2006): 1515, https://doi.org/10.1249/01.mss.0000227537.13175.1b.

25 Aaron Kandola et al., "Depressive Symptoms and Objectively Measured Physical Activity and Sedentary Behaviour throughout Adolescence: A Prospective Cohort Study," *Lancet Psychiatry* 7, no. 3 (2020): 262–71, https://doi.org/10.1016/S2215-0366(20)30034-1; Xihe Zhu, Justin A. Haegele, and Seán Healy, "Movement and Mental Health: Behavioral Correlates of Anxiety and Depression among Children of 6–17 Years Old in the US," *Mental Health and Physical Activity* 16 (2019): 60–65, https://doi.org/10.1016/j.mhpa.2019.04.002.

26 Diana Salas-Gomez et al., "Physical Activity Is Associated with Better Executive Function in University Students," *Frontiers in Human Neuroscience* 14 (2020): 11, https://doi.org/10.3389/fnhum.2020.00011.

27 Anne Herbert and Anna Esparham, "Mind–Body Therapy for Children with Attention-Deficit/Hyperactivity Disorder," *Children* 4, no. 5 (2017): 31, https://doi.org/10.3390%2Fchildren4050031.

28 Jeffrey J. Martin, Mitchell Craib, and Victoria Mitchell, "The Relationships of Anxiety and Self-Attention to Running Economy in Competitive Male Distance Runners," *Journal of Sports Sciences* 13, no. 5 (1995): 371–76, https://doi.org/10.1080/02640419508732252.

29 Yair Bar-Haim and Orit Bart, "Motor Function and Social Participation in Kindergarten Children," *Social Development* 15, no. 2 (2006): 296–310, https://onlinelibrary.wiley.com/doi/abs/10.1046/j.1467-9507.2006.00342.x; Sandra L. Hofferth and John F. Sandberg, "How American Children Spend Their Time," *Journal of Marriage and Family* 63, no. 2 (2001): 295–308, https://doi.org/10.1111/j.1741-3737.2001.00295.x.

30 Richard Louv, *Last Child in the Woods: Saving Our Children from Nature-Deficit Disorder* (Chapel Hill, NC: Algonquin Books, 2005).

31 Louv, *Last Child in the Woods*.

32 Gail F. Melson, *Why the Wild Things Are: Animals in the Lives of Children* (Cambridge, MA: Harvard University Press, 2001).

33 Jacqueline D. Goodway, Leah E. Robinson, and Heather Crowe, "Gender Differences in Fundamental Motor Skill Development in Disadvantaged Preschoolers from Two Geographical Regions," *Research Quarterly for Exercise and Sport* 81, no. 1 (2010): 17–24, https://doi.org/10.1080/02701367.2010.10599624.

34 Stuart Shanker, *Self-Reg: How to Help Your Child (and You) Break the Stress Cycle and Successfully Engage with Life* (New York: Penguin, 2016).

35 Adam J. Starr et al., "Symptoms of Posttraumatic Stress Disorder after Orthopaedic Trauma," *Journal of Bone and Joint Surgery* 86, no. 6 (2004): 1115–21, https://doi.org/10.2106/00004623-200406000-00001.

36 Fogel, *Body Sense*.

37 Yishul Wei et al., "I Keep a Close Watch on this Heart of Mine: Increased Interoception in Insomnia," *Sleep* 39, no. 12 (2016): 2113–24, https://doi.org/10.5665/sleep.6308; Lisa Quadt, Hugo D. Critchley, and Sarah N. Garfinkel, "The Neurobiology of Interoception in Health and Disease," *Annals of the New York Academy of Sciences* 1428, no. 1 (2018): 112–28, https://doi.org/10.1111/nyas.13915.

38 Wei et al., "I Keep a Close Watch."

39 Karl Ebner and Nicolas Singewald, "Individual Differences in Stress Susceptibility and Stress Inhibitory Mechanisms," *Current Opinion in Behavioral Sciences* 14 (2017): 54–64, http://dx.doi.org/10.1016/j.cobeha.2016.11.016; Roma Pahwa et al., "Chronic Inflammation," StatPearls, updated November 20, 2020, https://www.ncbi.nlm.nih.gov/books/NBK493173/.

40 Cornelia Niessen et al., "Stop Thinking: An Experience Sampling Study on Suppressing Distractive Thoughts at Work," *Frontiers in Psychology* 11 (2020): 1616, https://doi.org/10.3389/fpsyg.2020.01616.

41 Lori Haase et al., "When the Brain Does Not Adequately Feel the Body: Links between Low Resilience and Interoception," *Biological Psychology* 113 (2016): 37–45, https://doi.org/10.1016/j.biopsycho.2015.11.004.

42 Nia Fogelman and Turhan Canli, "Early Life Stress, Physiology, and Genetics: A Review," *Frontiers in Psychology* 10 (August 2, 2019), https://doi.org/10.3389/fpsyg.2019.01668.

43 Christine Heim and Charles B. Nemeroff, "The Role of Childhood Trauma in the Neurobiology of Mood and Anxiety Disorders: Preclinical and Clinical Studies," *Biological Psychiatry* 49, no. 12 (2001): 1023–39, https://doi.org/10.1016/S0006-3223(01)01157-X.

44 Haase et al., "Brain Does Not Adequately Feel," 43.

45 Dario Grossi et al., "Altered Functional Connectivity of Interoception in Illness Anxiety Disorder," *Cortex* 86, (2017): 22–32, https://doi.org/10.1016/j.cortex.2016.10.018; Jason A. Avery et al., "Major Depressive Disorder Is Associated with Abnormal Interoceptive Activity and Functional Connectivity in the Insula," *Biological Psychiatry* 76, no. 3 (2014): 258–66, https://doi.org/10.1016/j.biopsych.2013.11.027; Jonathan Savitz and Neil A. Harrison, "Interoception and Inflammation in Psychiatric Disorders," *Biological Psychiatry: Cognitive Neuroscience and Neuroimaging* 3, no. 6 (2018): 514–24, https://doi.org/10.1016/j.bpsc.2017.12.011; Satoshi Umeda et al., "Prospective Memory Mediated by Interoceptive Accuracy: A Psychophysiological Approach," *Philosophical Transactions of the Royal Society B: Biological Sciences* 371, no. 1708 (2016): 20160005, https://doi.org/10.1098/rstb.2016.0005; Herbert and Pollatos, "Attenuated Interoceptive Sensitivity"; André Schulz and Claus Vögele, "Interoception and Stress," *Frontiers in Psychology* 6 (2015): 993, https://doi.org/10.3389/fpsyg.2015.00993.

46 Abby C. King et al., "The Relationship between Repressive and Defensive Coping Styles and Blood Pressure Responses in Healthy, Middle-Aged Men and Women," *Journal of Psychosomatic Research* 34, no. 4 (1990): 461–71, https://doi.org/10.1016/0022-3999(90)90070-k; John W. Burns, "The Role of Attentional Strategies in Moderating Links between Acute Pain Induction and Subsequent Psychological Stress: Evidence for Symptom-Specific Reactivity among Patients with Chronic Pain versus Healthy Nonpatients," *Emotion* 6, no. 2 (2006): 180, https://doi.org/10.1037/1528-3542.6.2.180; Huan Song et al., "Stress Related Disorders and Risk of Cardiovascular Disease: Population Based, Sibling Controlled Cohort Study," *BMJ* 365, (2019): 11255, https://doi.org/10.1136/bmj.l1255.

47 Samuel Brod et al., "'As Above, So Below': Examining the Interplay between Emotion and the Immune System," *Immunology* 143, no. 3 (2014): 311–18, https://doi.org/10.1111/imm.12341.

48 Kara Baskin, "I Have Clinical Anxiety. If the Coronavirus Scares You, This Might Help," *Boston Globe*, March 25, 2020, https://www.bostonglobe.com

/2020/03/25/magazine/i-have-clinical-anxiety-if-coronavirus-scares-you -this-might-help/.

49 Stefan Duschek et al., "The Contributions of Interoceptive Awareness to Cognitive and Affective Facets of Body Experience," *Journal of Individual Differences* 36, no. 2 (2015): 110–18, https://doi.org/10.1027/1614-0001 /a000165.

Chapter 2

1 This chapter, and the theme of this book about three states of ESA, is based on my own personal experiences, my clinical observations as an ESA practitioner of Rosen Method bodywork, and more importantly, on a three-part research study of Rosen Method practitioners' observations of their clients. This book, however, is not intended primarily for clinicians or practitioners but rather for anyone who wishes to access their own restorative ESA. The everyday examples and descriptions in this book are, however, based in well-grounded clinical and scientific research. For more information on my research on these three states, see Alan Fogel, "Three States of Embodied Self-Awareness in Rosen Method Bodywork: Part 1: Practitioner Observations of their Clients," *Rosen Method International Journal* 13, no. 1 (2020): 4–36, https://1xhdko41sric25njz22ditir-wpengine.netdna-ssl .com/wp-content/uploads/2020/02/FogelPart1February21NewFigure1 version2.pdf; Alan Fogel, "Three States of Embodied Self-Awareness in Rosen Method Bodywork: Part 2: Practitioner Observations of Their Own Experiences," *Rosen Method International Journal* 13, no. 1 (2020): 37–57, https://1xhdko41sric25njz22ditir-wpengine.netdna-ssl.com/wp-content /uploads/2020/02/FogelPart2FinalJan28version1.pdf; and Alan Fogel, "Three States of Embodied Self-Awareness in Rosen Method Bodywork: Part 3: Practitioner Post-Session Notes," *Rosen Method International Journal* 13, no 1, (2020):58–118,https://1xhdko41sric25njz22ditir-wpengine.netdna-ssl.com /wp-content/uploads/2020/02/FogelPart3FinalJan28.pdf.

2 Brother David Steindl-Rast, *The Way of Silence: Engaging the Sacred in Daily Life* (Cincinnati, OH: Franciscan Media, 1989); Shepherd, *Radical Wholeness*; Suzanne Scurlock-Durana, *Reclaiming Your Body* (Novato, CA: New World Library, 2017); Michael A. Singer, *The Untethered Soul: The Journey Beyond Yourself* (Oakland, CA: New Harbinger, 2007).

3 Oliver Grewe et al., "Emotions over Time: Synchronicity and Development of Subjective, Physiological, and Facial Affective Reactions to Music," *Emotion* 7, no. 4 (2007): 774, https://doi.org/10.1037/1528-3542.7.4.774.

4 Ian R. Kleckner et al., "Evidence for a Large-Scale Brain System Supporting Allostasis and Interoception in Humans," *Nature Human Behaviour* 1, no. 5 (2017): 1–14, https://doi.org/10.1038/s41562-017-0069; A. D. (Bud)

Craig, *How Do You Feel? An Interoceptive Moment with Your Neurobiological Self* (Princeton, NJ: Princeton University Press, 2014).

5 Beate M. Herbert et al., "Interoception across Modalities: On the Relationship between Cardiac Awareness and the Sensitivity for Gastric Functions," *PloS One* 7, no. 5 (2012): e36646, https://doi.org/10.1371/journal .pone.0036646, p. 7.

6 Luma Muhtadie et al., "Neuroanatomy of Expressive Suppression: The Role of the Insula," *Emotion* 21, no. 2 (2021), 405–18, https://doi.org/10.1037 /emo0000710.

7 David G. Andrewes and Lisanne M. Jenkins, "The Role of the Amygdala and the Ventromedial Prefrontal Cortex in Emotional Regulation: Implications for Post-Traumatic Stress Disorder," *Neuropsychology Review* (2019): 1–24, https://doi.org/10.1007/s11065-019-09398-4.

8 Fogel, *Body Sense*.

9 Craig, *How Do You Feel?*; Mahlega S. Hassanpour et al., "The Insular Cortex Dynamically Maps Changes in Cardiorespiratory Interoception," *Neuropsychopharmacology* 43, no. 2 (2018): 426–34, https://doi.org/10.1038 /npp.2017.154.

10 Marius V. Peelen and Paul E. Downing, "The Neural Basis of Visual Body Perception," *Nature Reviews Neuroscience* 8, no. 8 (2007): 636–48, https://doi.org /10.1038/nrn2195.

11 Olivier Walusinski, "Yawning: Unsuspected Avenue for a Better Understanding of Arousal and Interoception," *Medical Hypotheses* 67, no. 1 (2006): 6–14, https://doi.org/10.1016/j.mehy.2006.01.020.

12 Fogel, *Body Sense*.

13 Bigna Lenggenhager and Christophe Lopez, "Vestibular Contributions to the Sense of Body, Self, and Others," in *Open Mind*, ed. Thomas K. Metzinger and Jennifer M. Windt (Frankfurt am Main, Germany: Open Mind, 2015), 1–38.

14 Lenggenhager and Lopez.

15 Weronika Grantham, Ejgil Jespersen, and Maciej Płaszewski, "Dancing My Scoliosis: An Autoethnography of Healing from Bodily Doubt through Somatic Practices," *Qualitative Research in Sport, Exercise and Health* (February 16, 2020): 1–17, https://doi.org/10.1080/2159676X.2020.1724190, p. 6.

16 Grantham, Jespersen, and Płaszewski, 9–10.

17 Grantham, Jespersen, and Płaszewski, 12.

18 Fiona K. O'Neill, "Bodily Knowing as Uncannily Canny: Clinical and Ethical Significance," *Sociological Review* 56, no. s2 (2008): 216–32, https://doi.org /10.1111%2Fj.1467-954X.2009.00824.x.

19 Mariana Babo-Rebelo, Craig G. Richter, and Catherine Tallon-Baudry, "Neural Responses to Heartbeats in the Default Network Encode the Self in Spontaneous Thoughts," *Journal of Neuroscience* 36, no. 30 (2016): 7829–40, https://doi.org/10.1523/JNEUROSCI.0262-16.2016.

20 Craig, *How Do You Feel?*

21 Fogel, *Body Sense.*

22 Fogel, *Body Sense.*

23 C. Sue Carter, "Oxytocin Pathways and the Evolution of Human Behavior," *Annual Review of Psychology* 65 (2014): 17–39, https://doi.org/10.1146 /annurev-psych-010213-115110; Stephen W. Porges, "The Polyvagal Theory: Phylogenetic Substrates of a Social Nervous System," *International Journal of Psychophysiology* 42, no. 2 (2001): 123–46, https://doi.org/10.1016 /s0167-8760(01)00162-3.

24 Craig, *How Do You Feel?*; Emily R. Stern et al., "Neural Correlates of Interoception: Effects of Interoceptive Focus and Relationship to Dimensional Measures of Body Awareness," *Human Brain Mapping* 38, no. 12 (2017): 6068–82, https://doi.org/10.1002/hbm.23811.

25 Dario Grossi et al., "The Brain Network for Self-Feeling: A Symptom-Lesion Mapping Study," *Neuropsychologia* 63, (2014): 92–98, http://dx.doi.org /10.1016/j.neuropsychologia.2014.08.004.

26 Olga Pollatos and Rainer Schandry, "Emotional Processing and Emotional Memory Are Modulated by Interoceptive Awareness," *Cognition & Emotion* 22, no. 2 (2008): 272–87, https://doi.org/10.1080/02699930701357535; Georg Northoff, "From Emotions to Consciousness—A Neuro-phenomenal and Neuro-relational Approach," *Frontiers in Psychology* 3 (2012): 303, https://doi.org/10.3389/fpsyg.2012.00303.

27 Barnaby D. Dunn et al., "Listening to Your Heart: How Interoception Shapes Emotion Experience and Intuitive Decision Making," *Psychological Science* 21, no. 12 (2010): 1835–44, https://doi.org/10.1177/0956797610389191.

28 Liliana L. Luz et al., "Monosynaptic Convergence of Somatic and Visceral C-Fiber Afferents on Projection and Local Circuit Neurons in Lamina I: A Substrate for Referred Pain," *Pain* 156, no. 10 (2015): 2042, https://doi.org /10.1097/j.pain.0000000000000267. Another mechanism for referred pain symptoms is via connective tissue (e.g., fascia) that links muscle groups together in the body, creating a kind of chain reaction that spreads from one location to another; see Dong-Gyun Han, "The Other Mechanism of Muscular Referred Pain: The 'Connective Tissue' Theory," *Medical Hypotheses* 73, no. 3 (2009): 292–95, https://doi.org/10.1016/j.mehy.2009.02.040.

29 Lauri Nummenmaa et al., "Maps of Subjective Feelings," *Proceedings of the National Academy of Sciences* 115, no. 37 (2018): 9198–203, https://doi.org /10.1073/pnas.1807390115.

30 Craig, *How Do You Feel?*

31 George A. Michael et al., "My Heart Is in My Hands: The Interoceptive Nature of the Spontaneous Sensations Felt on the Hands," *Physiology & Behavior* 143 (2015): 113–20, https://doi.org/10.1016/j.physbeh.2015.02.030; Hassanpour et al., "Maps of Subjective Feelings."

Chapter 3

1 Fogel, *Body Sense*.

2 Thomas Pinna and Darren J. Edwards, "A Systematic Review of Associations between Interoception, Vagal Tone, and Emotional Regulation: Potential Applications for Mental Health, Wellbeing, Psychological Flexibility, and Chronic Conditions," *Frontiers in Psychology* 11 (2020), https://doi.org/10.3389/fpsyg.2020.01792.

3 Lisa Dale Miller, "The Ultimate Rx: Cutting through the Delusion of Self-Cherishing," in *Handbook of Mindfulness: Culture, Context, and Social Engagement*, ed. Ronald E. Purser, David Forbes, and Adam Burke (Cham, Switzerland: Springer, 2016), 337–52.

4 Craig, *How Do You Feel?*

5 Michiel van Elk et al., "The Neural Correlates of the Awe Experience: Reduced Default Mode Network Activity during Feelings of Awe," *Human Brain Mapping* 40, no. 12 (2019): 3561–74, https://doi.org/10.1002/hbm.24616; Adam B. Cohen, June Gruber, and Dacher Keltner, "Comparing Spiritual Transformations and Experiences of Profound Beauty," *Psychology of Religion and Spirituality* 2, no. 3 (2010): 127, https://doi.org/10.1037/a0019126.

6 Laura A. Maruskin, Todd M. Thrash, and Andrew J. Elliot, "The Chills as a Psychological Construct: Content Universe, Factor Structure, Affective Composition, Elicitors, Trait Antecedents, and Consequences," *Journal of Personality and Social Psychology* 103, no. 1 (2012) 135–57, https://doi.org/10.1037/a0028117; William Braud, "Experiencing Tears of Wonder-Joy: Seeing with the Heart's Eye," *Journal of Transpersonal Psychology* 33, no. 2 (2001): 99–112.

7 Van Elk et al., "Neural Correlates"; J. M. de Castro, "A Model of Enlightened/Mystical/Awakened Experience," *Psychology of Religion and Spirituality* 9, no. 1 (2017): 34–45, https://doi.org/10.1037/rel0000037.

8 Michelle N. Shiota et al., "Feeling Good: Autonomic Nervous System Responding in Five Positive Emotions," *Emotion* 11, no. 6 (2011): 1368–78, https://doi.org/10.1037/a0024278.

9 Melanie Rudd, Kathleen D. Vohs, and Jennifer Aaker, "Awe Expands People's Perception of Time, Alters Decision Making, and Enhances Well-Being," *Psychological Science* 23, no. 10 (2012): 1130–36, https://doi.org/10.1177/%2F0956797612438731.

10 Craig L. Anderson, Maria Monroy, and Davher Keltner, "Awe in Nature Heals: Evidence from Military Veterans, At-Risk Youth, and College Students," *Emotion* 18, no. 8 (2018): 1195–202, https://doi.org/10.1037/emo0000442.

11 Kazuki Sawada and Michio Nomura, "Influence of Positive and Threatened Awe on the Attitude toward Norm Violations," *Frontiers in Psychology* 11 (2020): 148, https://doi.org/10.3389/fpsyg.2020.00148.

12 Huanhuan Zhao et al., "Why Are People High in Dispositional Awe Happier? The Roles of Meaning in Life and Materialism," *Frontiers in Psychology* 10 (2019): 1208, https://doi.org/10.3389/fpsyg.2019.01208; Qihao Ji et al., "The Melody to Inspiration: The Effects of Awe-Eliciting Music on Approach Motivation and Positive Well-Being," *Media Psychology* (2019): 1–27, https://doi.org/10.1080/15213269.2019.1693402; Jing-Jing Li et al., "Why Awe Promotes Prosocial Behaviors? The Mediating Effects of Future Time Perspective and Self-Transcendence Meaning of Life," *Frontiers in Psychology* 10 (2019): 1140, https://doi.org/10.3389/fpsyg.2019.01140; Patty Van Cappellen and Vassilis Saroglou, "Awe Activates Religious and Spiritual Feelings and Behavioral Intentions," *Psychology of Religion and Spirituality* 4, no. 3 (2012): 223–36, https://doi.org/10.1037/a0025986; Rudd, Vohs, and Aaker, "Awe Expands People's Perception of Time."

13 Cythia Frantz et al., "There Is No 'I' in Nature: The Influence of Self-Awareness on Connectedness to Nature," *Journal of Environmental Psychology* 25, no. 4 (2005): 427–36, https://doi.org/10.1016/j.envp.2005.10.002; Shepherd, *Radical Wholeness.*

14 David Bryce Yaden et al., "The Varieties of Self-Transcendent Experience," *Review of General Psychology* 21, no. 2 (2017): 143–60, https://doi.org/10.1037%2Fgpr0000102.

15 Paul K. Piff et al., "Awe, the Small Self, and Prosocial Behavior," *Journal of Personality and Social Psychology* 108, no. 6 (2015): 883–99, https://doi.org/10.1037/pspi0000018; de Castro, "Enlightened/Mystical/Awakened Experience"; Yaden et al., "Varieties of Self-Transcendent Experience"; Frantz et al., "There Is No 'I' in Nature."

16 Virginia E. Sturm et al., "Big Smile, Small Self: Awe Walks Promote Prosocial Positive Emotions in Older Adults," *Emotion* (2020, advance online publication), https://doi.org/10.1037/emo0000876.

17 Laura M. Edinger-Schons, "Oneness Beliefs and Their Effect on Life Satisfaction," *Psychology of Religion and Spirituality* 12, no. 4 (2020): 428–39, https://doi.org/10.1037/rel0000259.

18 Paul Gilbert et al., "Feeling Safe and Content: A Specific Affect Regulation System? Relationship to Depression, Anxiety, Stress, and Self-Criticism," *Journal of Positive Psychology* 3, no. 3 (2008): 182–91, https://doi.org/10.1080/17439760801999461.

19 Joana Duarte and Jose Pinto-Gouveia, "Positive Affect and Parasympathetic Activity: Evidence for a Quadratic Relationship between Feeling Safe and Content and Heart Rate Variability," *Psychiatric Research* 257 (2017): 284–89, https://doi.org/10.1016/j.psychres.2017.07.077.

20 Graham Music, "Bringing Up the Bodies: Psyche-Soma, Body Awareness and Feeling at Ease," *British Journal of Psychotherapy* 31, no. 1 (2015): 4–19, https://doi.org/10.1111/bjp.12122.

21 Daniel Stern, *The Present Moment in Psychotherapy and Everyday Life* (New York: W. W. Norton, 2004).

22 Steindl-Rast, *Way of Silence*; Fogel, *Body Sense*.

23 Mark Solms and Jaak Panksepp, "The 'Id' Knows More than the 'Ego' Admits," in *The Feeling Brain: Selected Papers on Neuropsychoanalysis*, ed. Mark Solms (New York: Routledge, 2015), 143–96.

24 Fogel, *Body Sense*.

25 Katrin Sakreida et al., "Are Abstract Action Words Embodied? An fMRI Investigation at the Interface between Language and Motor Cognition," *Frontiers in Human Neuroscience* 7 (2013): 125, https://doi.org/10.3389/fnhum.2013.00125.

26 Kathleen A. Garrison et al., "Effortless Awareness: Using Real Time Neurofeedback to Investigate Correlates of Posterior Cingulate Cortex Activity in Meditators' Self-Report," *Frontiers in Human Neuroscience* 7 (2013): 440, https://doi.org/10.3389/fnhum.2013.00440.

27 Will Adams, "Revelatory Openness Wedded with the Clarity of Unknowing: Psychoanalytic Evenly Suspended Attention, Phenomenological Attitude, and Meditative Awareness," *Psychoanalysis and Contemporary Thought* 18 (1995): 463–94; Mark D. Epstein, "On the Neglect of Evenly Suspended Attention," *Journal of Transpersonal Psychology* 16 (1984): 193–205; Antoine Lutz et al., "Investigating the Phenomenological Matrix of Mindfulness-Related Practices from a Neurocognitive Perspective," *American Psychologist* 70, no. 7 (2015): 632–58, https://doi.org/10.1037/a0039585.

28 Li-Jun Ji et al., "Global Processing Makes People Happier than Local Processing," *Frontiers in Psychology* 10 (2019): 670, https://doi.org/10.3389/fpsyg.2019.00670.

29 Darby E. Saxbe et al., "The Embodiment of Emotion: Language Use during the Feeling of Social Emotions Predicts Cortical Somatosensory Activity," *Social Cognitive and Affective Neuroscience* 8, no. 7 (2013): 806–12, https://doi.org/10.1093/scan/nss075.

30 Rebecca J. Lepping et al., "Preferential Activation for Emotional Western Classical Music versus Emotional Environmental Sounds in Motor, Interoceptive, and Language Brain Areas," *Brain and Cognition* 136 (2019): 103593, https://doi.org/10.1016/j.bandc.2019.103593; Grewe et al., "Emotions over Time."

31 Anne D. Rust-D'Eye, "The Sounds of the Self: Voice and Emotion in Dance/Movement Therapy," *Body, Movement and Dance in Psychotherapy* 8, no. 2 (2013): 95–107, https://doi.org/10.1080/17432979.2013.771702.

32 Enzo Grossi, Giorgio Tavano Blessi, and Pier Luigi Sacco, "Magic Moments: Determinants of Stress Relief and Subjective Wellbeing from Visiting a Cultural Heritage Site," *Culture, Medicine, and Psychiatry* 43, no. 1 (2019): 4–24, https://doi.org/10.1007/s11013-018-9593-8; Amy M. Belfi et al.,

"Dynamics of Aesthetic Experience Are Reflected in the Default-Mode Network," *NeuroImage* 188 (2019): 584–97, https://doi.org/10.1016/j.neuroimage.2018.12.017; Brittany S. Cassidy and Angela H. Gutchess, "Structural Variation within the Amygdala and Ventromedial Prefrontal Cortex Predicts Memory for Impressions in Older Adults," *Frontiers in Psychology* 3 (2012): 319, https://doi.org/10.3389/fpsyg.2012.00319.

33 Fogel, *Body Sense.*

34 Cassidy and Gutchess, "Structural Variation within the Amygdala"; Elisa Ciaramelli and Giuseppe de Pellegrino, "Ventromedial Prefrontal Cortex and the Future of Morality," *Emotion Review* 3, no. 3 (2011): 308–9, https://doi.org/10.1177%2F1754073911402381; Arnaud D'Argembeau, "On the Role of the Ventromedial Prefrontal Cortex in Self-Professing: The Valuation Hypothesis," *Frontiers in Human Neuroscience* 7 (2013): 372, https://doi.org/10.3389/fnhum.2013.00372.

35 Norberto Eiji Nawa and Hiroshi Ando, "Effective Connectivity within the Ventromedial Prefrontal Cortex-Hippocampus-Amygdala Network during the Elaboration of Emotional Autobiographical Memories," *NeuroImage* 189 (2019): 316–28, https://doi.org/10.1016/j.neuroimage.2019.01.042.

36 Sam J. Maglio and Taly Reich, "Feeling Certain: Gut Choice, the True Self, and Attitude Certainty," *Emotion* 19, no. 5 (2019): 876–88, https://doi.org/10.1037/emo0000490.

37 Donald W. Winnicott, *The Maturational Processes and the Facilitating Environment* (New York: International Universities Press, 1960),144, 148.

38 Romila Singh and Jeffrey H. Greenhaus, "The Relation between Career Decision-Making Strategies and Person-Job Fit: A Study of Job Changers," *Journal of Vocational Behavior* 64, no. 1 (2004): 198–221, https://doi.org/10.1016/S0001-8791(03)00034-4, p. 207.

39 Vitor H. Pereira, Isabel Campos, and Nuno Sousa, "The Role of Autonomic Nervous System in Susceptibility and Resilience to Stress," *Current Opinion in Behavioral Sciences* 14 (2017): 102–7, https://doi.org/10.1016/j.cobeha.2017.01.003; Carter, "Oxytocin Pathways"; Porges, "Polyvagal Theory."

40 Paula G. Williams et al., "Openness to Experience and Stress Regulation," *Journal of Research in Personality* 43, no. 5 (2009): 777–84, https://doi.org/10.1016/j.jrp.2009.06.003.

41 Paraic S. O'Suilleabhain, Siobhan Howard, and Brian M. Hughes, "Openness to Experience and Stress Responsivity: An Examination of Cardiovascular and Underlying Hemodynamic Trajectories within an Acute Stress Exposure," *PLoS One* 13, no. 6 (2018): e0199221, https://doi.org/10.1371/journal.pone.0199221; Williams et al., "Openness to Experience."

42 Louise Chim et al., "Valuing Calm Enhances Enjoyment of Calming (vs. Exciting) Amusement Park Rides and Exercise," *Emotion* 18, no. 6 (2018): 805–18, https://doi.org/10.1037/emo0000348.

43 Adriana Espinosa and Selma Kadic-Maglajlic, "The Mediating Role of Health Consciousness in the Relation between Emotional Intelligence and Health Behaviors," *Frontiers in Psychology* 9 (2018): 2161, https://doi.org/10.3389/fpsyg.2018.02161. The best, most validated self-report measures of emotional and body awareness are excellent at distinguishing modulated ESA from dysregulated ESA. This means that these measures can discern when people are able to either think about or directly engage with felt experience, as compared to when people are stuck in rumination, pain, or avoidance of felt experience (see, for example, Wolf E. Mehling et al., "The Multidimensional Assessment of Interoceptive Awareness [MAIA]," *PLoS One* 7, no. 11 (2012): e48230, https://doi.org/10.1371/journal.pone.0048230). Aside from some measures of awe or spiritual experiences, however, it is more difficult to find a reliable standardized self-report measurement of restorative ESA. I'm not entirely certain about this, but when experiences are transformed into questionnaire items using words and sentences, the respondent must access the TPN network to think about the answer, which, as we now know, shuts down the networks for felt experience. Most likely the only reliable way to scientifically measure restorative states is by brain scans and physiological measures of the ANS.

44 Marianna Szabo and Peter F. Lovibond, "Worry Episodes and Perceived Problem Solving: A Diary-Based Approach," *Anxiety, Stress & Coping* 19, no. 2 (2006): 175–87, https://doi.org/10.1080/10615800600643562; Marianna Szabo and Peter F. Lovibond, "The Cognitive Content of Naturally Occurring Worry Episodes," *Cognitive Therapy and Research* 26 (2002): 167–77, https://doi.org/10.1023/A:1014565602111; John M. Malouff, Einar B. Thorsteinsson, and Nicola S. Schutte, "The Efficacy of Problem Solving Therapy in Reducing Mental and Physical Health Problems: A Meta-analysis," *Clinical Psychology Review* 27, no. 1 (2007): 46–57, https://doi.org/10.1016/j.cpr.2005.12.005; Melanie J. Edwards et al., "Thinking about Thinking about Pain: A Qualitative Investigation of Rumination in Chronic Pain," *Pain Management* 1, no. 4 (2011): 311–23, https://doi.org/10.2217/pmt.11.29.

45 Kayla Isaacs et al., "Psychological Resilience in U.S. Military Veterans: A 2-year, Nationally Representative Prospective Cohort Study," *Journal of Psychiatric Research* 84 (2017): 301–9, https://doi.org/10.1016/j.jpsychires.2016.10.017.

46 Maria Teresa Sanchez Lopez et al., "The Relationship between Perceived Emotional Intelligence and Risk Behaviour in the Setting of Health," *Escritos de Psicologia* 11, no. 3 (2018): 115–23, http://dx.doi.org/10.5231/psy.writ.2018.2712.

47 Rosanna G. Lea et al., "Does Emotional Intelligence Buffer the Effects of Acute Stress? A Systematic Review," *Frontiers in Psychology* 10 (2019): 810, https://doi.org/10.3389/fpsyg.2019.00810.

48 Daniel Longman, Jay T. Stock, and Jonathan C. K. Wells, "A Trade-Off between Cognitive and Physical Performance, with Relative Preservation of Brain Function," *Scientific Reports* 7, no. 1 (2017): 1–6, https://doi.org/10.1038/s41598-017-14186-2.

49 Larry D. Jamner, Gary E. Schwartz, and Hoyle Leigh, "The Relationship between Repressive and Defensive Coping Styles and Monocyte, Eosinophile, and Serum Glucose Levels: Support for the Opioid Peptide Hypothesis of Repression," *Psychosomatic Medicine* 50, no. 6 (1988): 567–75, https://journals.lww.com/psychosomaticmedicine/Citation/1988/11000/The_relationship_between_repressive_and_defensive.2.aspx; Candace B. Pert et al., "Neuropeptides and Their Receptors: A Psychosomatic Network," *Journal of Immunology* 135, no. 2 (1985): 820–26, https://www.jimmunol.org/content/135/2/820.

50 Pereira, Campos, and Sousa, "Autonomic Nervous System in Susceptibility"; Sabine Sonnentag and Charlotte Fritz, "Recovery from Job Stress: The Stressor-Detachment Model as an Integrative Framework," *Journal of Organizational Behavior* 36, no. S1 (2015): S72–S103, https://doi.org/10.1002/job.1924.

51 Kirstin Aschbacher et al., "Good Stress, Bad Stress and Oxidative Stress: Insights from Anticipatory Cortisol Reactivity," *Psychoneuroendocrinology* 38, no. 9 (2013): 1698–708, https://doi.org/10.1016/j.psyneuen.2013.02.004; Chun-Tung Li, Jiannong Cao, and Tim M. H. Li, "Eustress or Distress: An Empirical Study of Perceived Stress in Everyday College Life," in *Proceedings of the 2016 ACM International Joint Conference on Pervasive and Ubiquitous Computing: Adjunct*, 2016, pp. 109–17, https://dl.acm.org/doi/pdf/10.1145/2968219.2968309; Williams et al., "Openness to Experience."

52 Katarina Habe, Michele Biasutti, and Tanja Kajtna, "Flow and Satisfaction with Life in Elite Musicians and Top Athletes," *Frontiers in Psychology* 10 (2019): 698, https://doi.org/10.3389/fpsyg.2019.00698; Narayanan Kandasamy et al., "Interoceptive Ability Predicts Survival on a London Trading Floor," *Scientific Reports* 6, no. 1 (2016): 1–7, https://doi.org/10.1038/srep32986.

53 Lauren N. Forrest et al., "(Dis)connected: An Examination of Interoception in Individuals with Suicidality," *Journal of Abnormal Psychology* 124, no. 3 (2015): 754–63, https://doi.org/10.1037/abn0000074.

54 Kasra Moazzami et al., "Association between Mental Stress-Induced Inferior Frontal Cortex Activation and Angina in Coronary Artery Disease," *Circulation: Cardiovascular Imaging* 13, no. 8 (2020): e010710, https://doi.org/10.1161/CIRCIMAGING.120.010710.

55 Richard P. Fleet et al., "Panic Disorder in Emergency Department Chest Pain Patients: Prevalence, Comorbidity, Suicidal Ideation, and Physician Recognition," *American Journal of Medicine* 101, no. 4 (1996): 371–80, https://doi.org/10.1016/S0002-9343(96)00224-0.

56 Aaron J. Fisher and Michelle G. Newman, "Heart Rate and Autonomic Response to Stress after Experimental Induction of Worry versus Relaxation in Healthy, High-Worry, and Generalized Anxiety Disorder Individuals," *Biological Psychology* 93, no. 1 (2013): 65–74, https://doi.org/10.1016/j.biopsycho.2013.01.012; Stuart D. Rosen, "From Heart to Brain: The Genesis and Processing of Cardiac Pain," *Canadian Journal of Cardiology* 28, no. 2 (2012): S7–S19, https://doi.org/10.1016/j.cjca.2011.09.010; James K. Ruffle et al., "Visceral Pain Endophenotypes Associate to Intricate Subcortical Brain Morphological Differences Contingent on Differing Autonomic Physiology or Personality," *Gastroenterology* 154, no. 6 (2018): S155–56, https://doi.org/10.1016/S0016-5085(18)30935-1.

57 Tom Schonberg et al., "Decreasing Ventromedial Prefrontal Cortex Activity during Sequential Risk-Taking: An fMRI Investigation of the Balloon Analog Risk Task," *Frontiers in Neuroscience* 6 (2012): 80, https://doi.org/10.3389/fnins.2012.00080; Rebecca M. Shansky and Jennifer Lipps, "Stress-Induced Cognitive Dysfunction: Hormone-Neurotransmitter Interactions in the Prefrontal Cortex," *Frontiers in Human Neuroscience* 7 (2013): 123, https://doi.org/10.3389/fnhum.2013.00123.

58 Antonio Verdejo-Garcia, Luke Clark, and Barnaby D. Dunn, "The Role of Interoception in Addiction: A Critical Review," *Neuroscience & Biobehavioral Reviews* 36, no. 8 (2012): 1857–69, https://doi.org/10.1016/j.neubiorev.2012.05.007.

59 Andrea N. Niles and Aoife O'Donovan, "Comparing Anxiety and Depression to Obesity and Smoking as Predictors of Major Medical Illnesses and Somatic Symptoms," *Health Psychology* 38, no. 2 (2019): 172–81, https://doi.org/10.1037/hea0000707.

60 Craig, *How Do You Feel?*; Stern et al., "Neural Correlates of Interoception"; Jon Julius Frederickson, Irene Messina, and Alessandro Grecucci, "Dysregulated Anxiety and Dysregulating Defenses: Toward an Emotion Regulation Informed Dynamic Psychotherapy," *Frontiers in Psychology* 9 (2018): 2054, https://doi.org/10.3389/fpsyg.2018.02054.

61 Dario Grossi et al., "Altered Functional Connectivity of Interoception in Illness Anxiety Disorder," *Cortex* 86 (2017): 22–32, https://doi.org/10.1016/j.cortex.2016.10.018; Beate M. Herbert and Olga Pollatos, "The Body in the Mind: On the Relationship between Interoception and Embodiment," *Topics in Cognitive Science* 4, no. 4 (2012): 692–704, https://doi.org/10.1111/j.1756-8765.2012.01189.x; Sigrid Elsenbruch et al., "Patients with Irritable Bowel Syndrome Have Altered Emotional Modulation of Neural Responses

to Visceral Stimuli," *Gastroenterology* 139, no. 4 (2010): 1310–19, https://doi.org/10.1053/j.gastro.2010.06.054; Antonia V. Seligowski et al., "Emotion Regulation and Posttraumatic Stress Symptoms: A Meta-analysis," *Cognitive Behaviour Therapy* 44, no. 2 (2015): 87–102, https://doi.org/10.1080/16506073.2014.980753; Dominic A. Trevisan et al., "A Meta-analysis on the Relationship between Interoceptive Awareness and Alexithymia: Distinguishing Interoceptive Accuracy and Sensibility," *Journal of Abnormal Psychology* 128, no. 8 (2019): 765–76, https://doi.org/10.1037/abn0000454; Sophie Sowden et al., "The Specificity of the Link between Alexithymia, Interoception, and Imitation," *Journal of Experimental Psychology: Human Perception and Performance* 42, no. 11 (2016): 1687–92, https://doi.org/10.1037/xhp0000310; Celine Borg et al., "Attentional Focus on Subjective Interoceptive Experience in Patients with Fibromyalgia," *Brain and Cognition* 101 (2015): 35–43, https://doi.org/10.1016/j.bandc.2015.10.002; Christopher Harshaw, "Interoceptive Dysfunction: Toward an Integrated Framework for Understanding Somatic and Affective Disturbance in Depression," *Psychological Bulletin* 141, no. 2 (2015): 311–63, https://doi.org/10.1037/a0038101.

62 Christine Wiebking et al., "GABA in the Insula—A Predictor of the Neural Response to Interoceptive Awareness," *NeuroImage* 86 (2014): 10–18, https://doi.org/10.1016/j.neuroimage.2013.04.042; Jason A. Avery et al., "Major Depressive Disorder Is Associated with Abnormal Interoceptive Activity and Functional Connectivity in the Insula," *Biological Psychiatry* 76, no. 3 (2014): 258–66, https://doi.org/10.1016/j.biopsych.2013.11.027.

63 Vivien Ainley et al., "'Bodily Precision': A Predictive Coding Account of Individual Differences in Interoceptive Accuracy," *Philosophical Transactions of the Royal Society B: Biological Sciences* 371, no. 1708 (2016): 20160003, https://doi.org/10.1098/rstb.2016.0003; Camila Valenzuela-Moguillansky, Alejandro Reyes-Reyes, and Maria I. Gaete, "Exteroceptive and Interoceptive Body-Self Awareness in Fibromyalgia Patients," *Frontiers in Human Neuroscience* 11 (2017): 117, https://doi.org/10.3389/fnhum.2017.00117.

64 F. C. Jellesma et al., "Do I Feel Sadness, Fear or Both? Comparing Self-Reported Alexithymia and Emotional Task-Performance in Children with Many or Few Somatic Complaints," *Psychology & Health* 24, no. 8 (2009): 881–93, https://doi.org/10.1080/08870440801998970.

65 Michele Mattle et al., "Association of Dance-Based Mind-Motor Activities with Falls and Physical Function among Healthy Older Adults: A Systematic Review and Meta-analysis," *JAMA Network Open* 3, no. 9 (2020): e2017688, https://doi.org/10.1001/jamanetworkopen.2020.17688; Jan-Christoph Kattenstroth et al., "Six Months of Dance Intervention Enhances Postural, Sensorimotor, and Cognitive Performance in Elderly without Affecting Cardio-respiratory Functions," *Frontiers in Aging Neuroscience* 5 (2013): 5, https://doi.org/10.3389/fnagi.2013.00005.

66 Wendy Berry Mendes, "Weakened Links between Mind and Body in Older Age: The Case for Maturational Dualism in the Experience of Emotion," *Emotion Review* 2, no. 3 (2010): 240–44, https://doi.org/10.1177/1754073910364149; Jennifer K. MacCormack et al., "Aging Bodies, Aging Emotions: Interoceptive Differences in Emotion Representations and Self-Reports across Adulthood," *Emotion* 21, no. 2 (2021): 227–46, https://doi.org/10.1037/emo0000699.

67 Indira Garcia-Cordero et al., "Feeling, Learning from and Being Aware of Inner States: Interoceptive Dimensions in Neurodegeneration and Stroke," *Philosophical Transactions of the Royal Society B: Biological Sciences* 371, no. 1708 (2016): 20160006, https://doi.org/10.1098/rstb.2016.0006.

68 Judith K. Daniels et al., "Default Mode Alterations in Posttraumatic Stress Disorder Related to Early-Life Trauma: A Developmental Perspective," *Journal of Psychiatry & Neuroscience* 36, no. 1 (2011): 56–59, https://doi.org/10.1503/jpn.100050; Joachim Kowalski et al., "Neural Correlates of Cognitive-Attentional Syndrome: An fMRI Study on Repetitive Negative Thinking Induction and Resting State Functional Connectivity," *Frontiers in Psychology* 10 (2019): 648, https://doi.org/10.3389/fpsyg.2019.00648.

69 Stefanie M. Jungmann et al., "Understanding Dysregulated Behaviors and Compulsions: An Extension of the Emotional Cascade Model and the Mediating Role of Intrusive Thoughts," *Frontiers in Psychology* 7 (2016): 994, https://doi.org/10.3389/fpsyg.2016.00994; Tabea Flasinski et al., "Altered Interoceptive Awareness in High Habitual Symptom Reporters and Patients with Somatoform Disorders," *Frontiers in Psychology* 11 (2020), 1859, https://doi.org/10.3389/fpsyg.2020.01859.

70 Ha Rin Kwon, Yookyung Eoh, and Soo Hyun Park, "The Mediating Role of Catastrophizing in the Relationship between Emotional Clarity and Posttraumatic Stress Symptoms among Earthquake Survivors in Korea: A Cross-Sectional Study," *Frontiers in Psychology* 11 (2020), 1114, https://doi.org/10.3389/fpsyg.2020.01114.

71 Heim and Nemeroff, "Role of Childhood Trauma."

72 Lihong Wang et al., "Loss of Sustained Activity in the Ventromedial Prefrontal Cortex in Response to Repeated Stress in Individuals with Early-Life Emotional Abuse: Implications for Depression Vulnerability," *Frontiers in Psychology* 4 (2013): 320, https://doi.org/10.3389/fpsyg.2013.00320; Heledd Hart and Katya Rubia, "Neuroimaging of Child Abuse: A Critical Review," *Frontiers in Human Neuroscience* 6 (2012): 52, https://doi.org/10.3389/fnhum.2012.00052; Allan N. Schore, *Affect Dysregulation and Disorders of the Self* (New York: W. W. Norton, 2003).

73 Sung W. Lee et al., "A Bihemispheric Autonomic Model for Traumatic Stress Effects on Health and Behavior," *Frontiers in Psychology* 5 (2014): 843, https://doi.org/10.3389/fpsyg.2014.00843; Pereira, Campos, and Sousa,

"Autonomic Nervous System in Susceptibility"; Schulz and Vögele, "Interoception and Stress."

74 Katleen Bogaerts et al., "Hyperventilation in Patients with Chronic Fatigue Syndrome: The Role of Coping Strategies," *Behaviour Research and Therapy* 45, no. 11 (2007): 2679–90, https://doi.org/10.1016/j.brat.2007.07.003; Janine Thome et al., "Desynchronization of Autonomic Response and Central Autonomic Network Connectivity in Posttraumatic Stress Disorder," *Human Brain Mapping* 38, no. 1 (2017): 27–40, https://doi.org /10.1002/hbm.23340; Frederickson, Messina, and Grecucci, "Dysregulated Anxiety and Dysregulating Defenses"; Christiane A. Melzig et al., "Interoceptive Threat Leads to Defensive Mobilization in Highly Anxiety Sensitive Persons," *Psychophysiology* 48, no. 6 (2011): 745–54, https://doi.org /10.1111/j.1469-8986.2010.01150.x.

75 Jonathan S. A. Carriere et al., "Wandering in Both Mind and Body: Individual Differences in Mind Wandering and Inattention Predict Fidgeting," *Canadian Journal of Experimental Psychology* 67, no. 1 (2013): 19–31, https://doi .org/10.1037/a0031438; David Stawarczyk et al., "Using the Daydreaming Frequency Scale to Investigate the Relationships between Mind-Wandering, Psychological Well-Being, and Present-Moment Awareness," *Frontiers in Psychology* 3 (2012): 363, https://doi.org/10.3389/fpsyg.2012.00363.

76 Nicholas Medford et al., "Emotional Memory in Depersonalization Disorder: A Functional MRI Study," *Psychiatry Research: Neuroimaging* 148, no. 2–3 (2006): 93–102, https://doi.org/10.1016/j.pscychresns.2006.05.007.

77 Vittorio Lenzo et al., "A Systematic Review of Metacognitive Beliefs in Chronic Medical Conditions," *Frontiers in Psychology* 10 (2019): 2875, https://doi.org /10.3389/fpsyg.2019.02875; Martin P. Paulus and Murray B. Stein, "Interoception in Anxiety and Depression," *Brain Structure and Function* 214 (2010): 451–63, https://doi.org/10.1007/s00429-010-0258-9; Herbert and Pollatos, "Body in the Mind"; Valenzuela-Moguillansky, Reyes-Reyes, and Gaete, "Body-Self Awareness in Fibromyalgia."

78 Edward A. Selby, Michael D. Anestis, and Thomas E. Joiner, "Understanding the Relationship between Emotional and Behavioral Dysregulation: Emotional Cascades," *Behaviour Research and Therapy* 46, no. 5 (2008): 593–611, https://doi.org/10.1016/j.brat.2008.02.002; Claire E. Wilcox, Jessica M. Pommy, and Byron Adinoff, "Neural Circuitry of Impaired Emotion Regulation in Substance Use Disorders," *American Journal of Psychiatry* 173, no. 4 (2016): 344–61, https://doi.org/10.1176/appi.ajp.2015.15060710.

79 Anne Kever et al., "The Body Language: The Spontaneous Influence of Congruent Bodily Arousal on the Awareness of Emotional Words," *Journal of Experimental Psychology: Human Perception and Performance* 41, no. 3 (2015): 582–89, https://doi.org/10.1037/xhp0000055.

80 Stefan Duschek et al., "The Contributions of Interoceptive Awareness to Cognitive and Affective Facets of Body Experience," *Journal of Individual Differences* 36 (2015): 110–18, https://doi.org/10.1027/1614-0001/a000165.

Chapter 4

1 Rudolph Bauer, "Transitional Space: An Opening of the Experiential Realm beyond the Mind: A Phenomenology," *Transmission* 8 (2017), https://www.journalofawareness.com/post/transitional-space-an-opening-of-the-experiential-realm-beyond-the-mind-a-phenomenology.

2 Stefon J. R. van Noordt and Signey J. Segalowitz, "Performance Monitoring and the Medial Prefrontal Cortex: A Review of Individual Differences and Context Effects as a Window on Self-Regulation," *Frontiers in Human Neuroscience* 6 (2012): 197, https://doi.org/10.3389/fnhum.2012.00197.

3 Marina Dyskant Mochcovitch et al., "A Systematic Review of fMRI Studies in Generalized Anxiety Disorder: Evaluating Its Neural and Cognitive Basis," *Journal of Affective Disorders* 167, no. 1 (2014): 336–42, https://doi.org/10.1016/j.jad.2014.06.041; M. Justin Kim et al., "The Structural and Functional Connectivity of the Amygdala: From Normal Emotion to Pathological Anxiety," *Behavioural Brain Research* 223, no. 2 (2011): 403–10, https://doi.org/10.1016/j.bbr.2011.04.025.

4 Annie T. Ginty et al., "Ventromedial Prefrontal Cortex Connectivity during and after Psychological Stress in Women," *Psychophysiology* 56, no. 11 (2019): e13445, https://doi.org/10.1111/psyp.13445.

5 Cassidy and Gutchess, "Structural Variation within the Amygdala."

6 Arnaud D'Argembeau, "On the Role of the Ventromedial Prefrontal Cortex in Self-Processing: The Valuation Hypothesis," *Frontiers in Human Neuroscience* 7 (2013): 372, https://doi.org/10.3389/fnhum.2013.00372.

7 Wang et al., "Loss of Sustained Activity."

8 Schonberg et al., "Decreasing Ventromedial Prefrontal Cortex Activity."

9 Randy L. Buckner, Jessica R. Andrews-Hanna, and Daniel L. Schacter, "The Brain's Default Network: Anatomy, Function, and Relevance to Disease," *Annals of the New York Academy of Sciences* 1124, no. 1 (2008): 1–38, https://doi.org/10.1196/annals.1440.011.

10 Esther Via et al., "Ventromedial Prefrontal Cortex Activity and Pathological Worry in Generalised Anxiety Disorder," *British Journal of Psychiatry* 213, no. 1 (2018): 437–43, https://doi.org/10.1192/bjp.2018.65; Eva-Maria Seidel et al., "Neural Correlates of Depressive Realism—An fMRI Study on Causal Attribution in Depression," *Journal of Affective Disorders* 138, no. 3 (2012): 268–76, https://doi.org/10.1016/j.jad.2012.01.041.

11 Martina Amanzio et al., "Executive Dysfunction and Reduced Self-Awareness in Patients with Neurological Disorders. A Mini-Review," *Frontiers in Psychology* 11 (2020): 1697, https://doi.org/10.3389/fpsyg.2020.01697.

12 Edmund T. Rolls, "The Functions of the Orbitofrontal Cortex," *Brain and Cognition* 55, no. 1 (2004): 11–29, https://doi.org/10.1016/S0278-2626(03)00277-X.

13 Valerie T. Chang et al., "Expressive Suppression Tendencies, Projection Bias in Memory of Negative Emotions, and Well-Being," *Emotion* 18, no. 7 (2018): 925–41, https://doi.org/10.1037/emo0000405; Siqi Fang, Man Cheung Chung, and Yabing Wang, "The Impact of Past Trauma on Psychological Distress: The Roles of Defense Mechanisms and Alexithymia," *Frontiers in Psychology* 11 (2020): 992, https://doi.org/10.3389/fpsyg.2020.00992.

14 Shansky and Lipps, "Stress-Induced Cognitive Dysfunction."

15 Paula G. Williams, Yana Suchy, and Holly K. Rau, "Individual Differences in Executive Functioning: Implications for Stress Regulation," *Annals of Behavioral Medicine* 37, no. 2 (2009): 126–40, https://doi.org/10.1007/s12160-009-9100-0; Vanessa M. Brown and Rajendra A. Morey, "Neural Systems for Cognitive and Emotional Processing in Posttraumatic Stress Disorder," *Frontiers in Psychology* 3 (2012): 449, https://doi.org/10.3389/fpsyg.2012.00449.

16 Mark E. Czeisler et al., "Mental Health, Substance Use, and Suicidal Ideation during the COVID-19 Pandemic—United States, June 24–30, 2020," *Morbidity and Mortality Weekly Report* 69, no. 32 (2020): 1049–57, https://doi.org/10.15585/mmwr.mm6932a1, p. 1053.

17 Mark Epstein, "The Trauma of Being Alive," *New York Times*, August 3, 2013, https://nyti.ms/17/qzT60.

18 Bessel van der Kolk, *The Body Keeps the Score: Brain, Mind and Body in the Healing of Trauma* (New York: Penguin Books, 2014); Peter A. Levine, *Waking the Tiger: Healing Trauma* (Berkeley, CA: North Atlantic Books, 1997); Pat Ogden, Kekuni Minton, and Clare Pain, *Trauma and the Body: A Sensorimotor Approach to Psychotherapy* (New York: W. W. Norton, 2006); Porges, "Polyvagal Theory."

19 Van der Kolk, *Body Keeps the Score*.

20 Steven C. Hayes et al., "Experiential Avoidance and Behavioral Disorders: A Functional Dimensional Approach to Diagnosis and Treatment," *Journal of Consulting and Clinical Psychology* 64, no. 6 (1996): 1152–68, https://doi.org/10.1037/0022-006X.64.6.1152, p. 1154.

21 Patrice Duquette, "More than Words Can Say: A Multi-disciplinary Consideration of the Psychotherapeutic Evaluation and Treatment of Alexithymia," *Frontiers in Psychiatry* 11 (2020): 433, https://doi.org/10.3389/fpsyt.2020.00433.

22 Duquette, "More than Words Can Say," 433; Patrice Duquette and Vivien Ainley, "Working with the Predictable Life of Patients: The Importance of 'Mentalizing Interoception' to Meaningful Change in Psychotherapy," *Frontiers in Psychology* 10 (2019): 2173, https://doi.org/10.3389/fpsyg.2019.02173; Hugo D. Critchley and Neil A. Harrison, "Visceral Influences on Brain and Behavior," *Neuron* 77, no. 4 (2013): 624–38, https://doi.org/10.1016/j.neuron.2013.02.008.

23 Caitlin McLean and Victoria M. Follette, "Acceptance and Commitment Therapy as a Nonpathologizing Intervention Approach for Survivors of Trauma," *Journal of Trauma & Dissociation* 17, no. 2 (2016): 138–50, https://doi.org/10.1080/15299732.2016.1103111.

24 McLean and Follette.

25 McLean and Follette.

26 Fogel, "Practitioner Observations of Their Clients."

27 McLean and Follette.

28 Fogel, *Body Sense*; Fogel, "Practitioner Observations of Their Clients"; Anais Salibian, "Trauma Therapy with Rosen Method Bodywork," *Rosen Method International Journal* 8, no. 1 (2015): 4–33, https://1xhdko41sric25njz22ditir-wpengine.netdna-ssl.com/wp-content/uploads/2015/06/2015-vol8iss1-2.pdf; Ivy Green, "Attachment Patterns and Emotion Regulation in Interpersonal Relationships," *Rosen Method International Journal* 7, no. 1 (2014): 30–48, https://1xhdko41sric25njz22ditir-wpengine.netdna-ssl.com/wp-content/uploads/2015/06/2014-vol7iss1-3.pdf.

29 Elizabeth A. Behnke, "The Study Project in Phenomenology of the Body," *Humanistic Psychologist* 22, no. 3 (1994): 296–17, https://doi.org/10.1080/08873267.1994.9976956, pp. 305–6.

30 Elizabeth H. Eustis et al., "Reductions in Experiential Avoidance as a Mediator of Change in Symptom Outcome and Quality of Life in Acceptance-Based Behavior Therapy and Applied Relaxation for Generalized Anxiety Disorder," *Behaviour Research and Therapy* 87 (2016): 188–95, https://doi.org/10.1016/j.brat.2016.09.012.

31 Merete Holm Brantbjerg, "Hyporesponse: The Hidden Challenge in Coping with Stress," *International Body Psychotherapy Journal* 11, no. 2 (2012): 95–118, https://www.ibpj.org/issues/articles/Holm%20Brantbjerg%20-%20Hyporesponse.pdf, pp. 107–8.

32 Peter Payne, Peter A. Levine, and Mardi A. Crane-Godreau, "Somatic Experiencing: Using Interoception and Proprioception as Core Elements of Trauma Therapy," *Frontiers in Psychology* 6 (2015): 93, https://doi.org/10.3389/fpsyg.2015.00093.

33 Edward C. Suarez et al., "Increases in Stimulated Secretion of Proinflammatory Cytokines by Blood Monocytes Following Arousal of Negative Affect:

The Role of Insulin Resistance as Moderator," *Brain, Behavior, and Immunity* 20, no. 4 (2006): 331–38, https://doi.org/10.1016/j.bbi.2005.09.005.

Chapter 5

1 Ian R. Kleckner et al., "Evidence for a Large-Scale Brain System Supporting Allostasis and Interoception in Humans," *Nature Human Behaviour* 1, no. 5 (2017): 1–14, https://doi.org/10.1038/s41562-017-0069.
2 Mike Osborn and Jonathan A. Smith, "Living with a Body Separate from the Self. The Experience of the Body in Chronic Benign Low Back Pain: An Interpretative Phenomenological Analysis," *Scandinavian Journal of Caring Science* 20, no. 2 (2006): 216–22, https://doi:.org/10.1111/j.1471-6712.2006.00399.x.
3 Phillip J. Quartana, John W. Burns, and Kenneth R. Lofland, "Attentional Strategy Moderates Effects of Pain Catastrophizing on Symptom-Specific Physiological Responses in Chronic Low Back Pain Patients," *Journal of Behavioral Medicine* 30, no. 3 (2007): 221–31, https://doi.org/10.1007/s10865-007-9101-z; Henriet van Middendorp et al., "Emotions and Emotional Approach and Avoidance Strategies in Fibromyalgia," *Journal of Psychosomatic Research* 64, no. 2 (2008): 159–67, https://doi.org/10.1016/j.psychores.2007.08.009.
4 Adrienne Levy Berg, Christer Sandahl, and Jennifer Bullington, "Patients' Perspective of Change Processes in Affect-Focused Body Psychotherapy for Generalised Anxiety Disorder," *Body, Movement and Dance in Psychotherapy* 5, no. 2 (2010): 151–69, https://doi.org/10.1080/17432979.2010.494853.
5 Berg, Sandahl, and Bullington, 160.
6 Berg, Sandahl, and Bullington, 161.
7 Berg, Sandahl, and Bullington, 162.
8 Wolf E. Mehling et al., "Body Awareness: A Phenomenological Inquiry into the Common Ground of Mind-Body Therapies," *Philosophy, Ethics, and Humanities in Medicine* 6, no. 1 (2011): 6, https://doi.org/10.1186/1747-5341-6-6, p. 8.
9 Mehling et al., 9.
10 Mehling et al., 9.
11 Mehling et al., 10.
12 Elsa M. Eriksson et al., "Body Awareness Therapy: A New Strategy for Relief of Symptoms in Irritable Bowel Syndrome Patients," *World Journal of Gastroenterology* 13, no. 23 (2007): 3206–14, https://doi.org/10.3748/wjg.v13.i23.3206.
13 Fogel, "Practitioner Observations of Their Clients."
14 Alan Fogel, "Better or Worse: A Study of Day-to-Day Changes over Five Months of Rosen Method Bodywork Treatment for Chronic Low Back Pain,"

International Journal of Therapeutic Massage & Bodywork 6, no. 3 (2013): 14–24, https://doi.org/10.3822/ijtmb.v6i3.200.

15 C. Richard Chapman and Yoshio Nakamura, "Pain and Consciousness: A Constructivist Approach," *Pain Forum* 8, no. 3 (1999): 113–23, https://doi.org /10.1016/S1082-3174(99)70019-X.

16 Sandra Manninen et al., "Social Laughter Triggers Endogenous Opioid Release in Humans," *Journal of Neuroscience* 37, no. 25 (2017): 6125–31, https://doi.org/10.1523/JNEUROSCI.0688-16.2017; Robin I. M. Dunbar et al., "Social Laughter Is Correlated with an Elevated Pain Threshold," *Proceedings of the Royal Society B: Biological Sciences* 279, no. 1731 (2012): 1161–67, https://doi.org/10.1098/rspb.2011.1373.

17 Avi Steinberg, "The Connoisseur of Pain," *New York Times,* August 8, 2016, https://nyti.ms/2bkAHmF.

18 Kirsten Weir, "The Pain of Social Rejection," *Monitor on Psychology* 43, no. 4 (2012): 50, https://www.apa.org/monitor/2012/04/rejection; Ethan Kross et al., "Social Rejection Shares Somatosensory Representations with Physical Pain," *Proceedings of the National Academy of Sciences* 108, no. 15 (2011): 6270–75, https://doi.org/10.1073/pnas.1102693108.

19 Kross et al.; Naomi I. Eisenberger, Matthew D. Lieberman, and Kipling D. Williams, "Does Rejection Hurt? An fMRI Study of Social Exclusion," *Science* 302, no. 5643 (2003): 290–92, https://doi.org/10.1126/science.1089134.

20 Neil A. Harrison et al., "The Embodiment of Emotional Feelings in the Brain," *Journal of Neuroscience* 30, no. 38 (2010): 12878–84, https://doi.org /10.1523/JNEUROSCI.1725-10.2010.

21 Tracy H. Wang, Katerina Placek, and Jarrod A. Lewis-Peacock, "More Is Less: Increased Processing of Unwanted Memories Facilitates Forgetting," *Journal of Neuroscience* 39, no. 18 (2019): 3551–60, https://doi.org/10.1523 /JNEUROSCI.2033-18.2019.

22 Judith Meessen et al., "The Relationship Between Interoception and Metacognition: A Pilot Study," *Journal of Psychophysiology* 30, (2016): 76–86, https://doi.org/10.1027/0269-8803/a000157.

23 Paul M. Jenkinson, Lauren Taylor, and Keith R. Laws, "Self-Reported Interoceptive Deficits in Eating Disorders: A Meta-analysis of Studies Using the Eating Disorder Inventory," *Journal of Psychosomatic Research* 110 (2018): 38–45, https://doi.org/10.1016/j.jpsychores.2018.04.005; Olga Pollatos et al., "Reduced Perception of Bodily Signals in Anorexia Nervosa," *Eating Behaviors* 9, no. 4 (2008): 381–88, https://doi.org/10.1016/j.eatbeh.2008.02.001; Marjo J. S. Zonnevylle-Bender et al., "Adolescent Anorexia Nervosa Patients Have a Discrepancy between Neurophysiological Responses and Self-Reported Emotional Arousal to Psychosocial Stress," *Psychiatry Research* 135, no. 1 (2005): 45–52, https://doi.org/10.1016/j.psychres.2004 .11.006.

24 Sonja Spoor et al., "Inner Body and Outward Appearance: The Relationships between Appearance Orientation, Eating Disorder Symptoms, and Internal Body Awareness," *Eating Disorders* 13, no. 5 (2005): 479–90, https://doi.org /10.1080/10640260500297267.

25 Erin Barker, Rebecca Williams, and Nancy Galambos, "Daily Spillover to and from Binge Eating in First-Year University Females," *Eating Disorders* 14, no. 3 (2006): 229–42, https://doi.org/10.1080/10640260600639079.

26 Sabine Frank, Stephanie Kullmann, and Ralf Veit, "Food Related Processes in the Insular Cortex," *Frontiers in Human Neuroscience* 7 (2013): 499, https:// doi.org/10.3389/fnhum.2013.00499.

27 Johan Vanderlinden et al., "Dissociative Experiences and Trauma in Eating Disorders," *International Journal of Eating Disorders* 13, no. 2 (1993): 187–93, https://doi.org/10.1002/1098-108x(199303)13:2%3C187::aid -eat2260130206%3E3.0.co;2-9; Sefik Tagay et al., "Eating Disorders, Trauma, PTSD and Psychosocial Resources," *Eating Disorders* 22, no. 1 (2014): 33–49, https://doi.org/10.1080/10640266.2014.857517.

28 Susanne Ohmann and Christian Popow, "Self Injurious Behavior in Adolescent Girls with Eating Disorders," in *Relevant Topics in Eating Disorders*, ed. Ignacio Jauregui Lobera (London: InTech Europe, 2012), 133–62, https:// doi.org/10.5772/31857.

29 Tamas Treuer et al., "The Impact of Physical and Sexual Abuse on Body Image in Eating Disorders," *European Eating Disorders Review* 13, no. 2 (2005): 106–11, https://doi.org/10.1002/erv.616.

30 Jason M. Nagata et al., "Predictors of Muscularity-Oriented Disordered Eating Behaviors in U.S. Young Adults: A Prospective Cohort Study," *International Journal of Eating Disorders* 52, no. 12 (2019): 1380–88, https://doi.org /10.1002/eat.23094.

31 Payton, "Bodies under Siege"; Jason M. Nagata et al., "Gender Norms and Weight Control Behaviors in U.S. Adolescents: A Prospective Cohort Study (1994–2002)," *Journal of Adolescent Health* 66, no. 1 (2020): S34–S41, https://doi.org/10.1016/j.jadohealth.2019.08.020.

32 Helga Dittmar, Emma Halliwell, and Suzanne Ive, "Does Barbie Make Girls Want to Be Thin? The Effect of Experimental Exposure to Images of Dolls on the Body Image of 5- to 8-year-old Girls," *Developmental Psychology* 42, no. 2 (2006): 283–92, https://doi.org/10.1037/0012-1649.42.2.283.

33 Tracy L. Dunkley, Eleanor H. Wertheim, and Susan J. Paxton, "Examination of a Model of Multiple Sociocultural Influences on Adolescent Girls' Body Dissatisfaction and Dietary Restraint," *Adolescence* 36, no. 142 (2001): 265–79, https://pubmed.ncbi.nlm.nih.gov/11572305/; Sarah Kate Beaman et al., "The Skinny on Body Dissatisfaction: A Longitudinal Study of Adolescent Girls and Boys," *Journal of Youth and Adolescence* 35, no. 2 (2006): 217–29, https://doi.org/10.1007/s10964-005-9010-9.

34 Julie J. Exline et al., "People-Pleasing through Eating: Sociotropy Predicts Greater Eating in Response to Perceived Social Pressure," *Journal of Social and Clinical Psychology* 31, no. 2, (2012): 169–93, https://doi.org/10.1521/jscp.2012.31.2.169.

35 Camilla Matera, A. Nerini, and C. Stefanile, "The Role of Peer Influence on Girls' Body Dissatisfaction and Dieting," *European Review of Applied Psychology* 63, no. 2 (2013): 67–74, https://doi.org/10.1016/j.erap.2012.08.002; Tiffany A. Meyer and Julie Gast, "The Effects of Peer Influence on Disordered Eating Behavior," *Journal of School Nursing* 24, no. 1 (2008) 36–42, https://doi.org/10.1177/10598405080240010601; Eric Stice and Kathryn Whitenton, "Risk Factors for Body Dissatisfaction in Adolescent Girls: A Longitudinal Investigation," *Developmental Psychology* 38, no. 5 (2002): 669–78, https://doi.org/10.1037/0012-1649.38.5.669.

36 Patricia Barthalow Koch et al., "'Feeling Frumpy': The Relationships between Body Image and Sexual Response Changes in Midlife Women," *Journal of Sex Research* 42, no. 3 (2005): 215–23, https://doi.org/10.1080/00224490509552276.

37 Anne M. Haase, Victoria Mountford, and Glenn Waller, "Understanding the Link between Body Checking Cognitions and Behaviors: The Role of Social Physique Anxiety," *International Journal of Eating Disorders* 40, no. 3 (2007): 241–46, https://doi.org/10.1002/eat.20356.

38 Jeffrey A. Katula and Edward McAuley, "The Mirror Does Not Lie: Acute Exercise and Self-Efficacy," *International Journal of Behavioral Medicine* 8, no. 4 (2001): 319–26, https://doi.org/10.1207/s15327558ijbm0804_6; Thomas G. Plante et al., "The Influence of Exercise Environment and Gender on Mood and Exertion," *International Journal of Exercise Science* 7, no. 3 (2014): 220–27, https://www.ncbi.nlm.nih.gov/pmc/articles/PMC4831862/.

39 Diana Taut, Britta Renner, and Adriana Baban, "Reappraise the Situation but Express Your Emotions: Impact of Emotion Regulation Strategies on Ad Libitum Food Intake," *Frontiers in Psychology* 3 (2012): 359, https://doi.org/10.3389/fpsyg.2012.00359.

40 Beate M. Herbert et al., "Intuitive Eating Is Associated with Interoceptive Sensitivity. Effects on Body Mass Index," *Appetite* 70, no. 1 (2013): 22–30, https://doi.org/10.1016/j.appet.2013.06.082.

41 Klazine van der Horst, "Overcoming Picky Eating. Eating Enjoyment as a Central Aspect of Children's Eating Behaviors," *Appetite* 58, no. 2 (2012): 567–74, https://doi.org/10.1016/j.appet.2011.12.019.

42 Michael Pollan, *The Omnivore's Dilemma: A Natural History of Four Meals* (Penguin Books, 2006).

43 Barbara H. Fiese and Marlene Schwartz, "Reclaiming the Family Table: Mealtimes and Child Health and Wellbeing," *Social Policy Report* 22, no. 4 (2008): 1–20, https://doi.org/10.1002/j.2379-3988.2008.tb00057.x.

44 Slow Food International, https://www.slowfood.com/.

45 Sarah E. Jackson et al., "Is There a Relationship between Chocolate Consumption and Symptoms of Depression? A Cross-Sectional Survey of 13,626 US Adults," *Depression & Anxiety* 36, no. 10 (2019): 987–95, https://doi.org/10.1002/da.22950.

46 Mark Epstein, *Thoughts without a Thinker* (New York: Basic Books, 1995), 148–49.

47 Shane McIver, Michael McGartland, and Paul O'Halloran, "Overeating Is Not about the Food. Women Describe Their Experience of a Yoga Treatment Program for Binge Eating," *Qualitative Health Research* 19, no. 9 (2009): 1234–45, https://doi.org/10.1177/1049732309343954.

48 McIver, McGartland, and O'Halloran, 1238.

49 Jean L. Kristeller and Kevin D. Jordan, "Mindful Eating: Connecting with the Wise Self, the Spiritual Self," *Frontiers in Psychology* 9 (2018): 1271, https://doi.org/10.3389/fpsyg.2018.01271, p. 9.

50 McIver, McGartland, and O'Halloran, "Overeating," 1238.

51 Angela Kong et al., "Self-Monitoring and Eating-Related Behaviors Are Associated with 12-Month Weight Loss in Postmenopausal Overweight-to-Obese Women," *Journal of the Academy of Nutrition and Dietetics* 112, no. 9 (2012): 1428–35, https://doi.org/10.1016/j.jand.2012.05.014.

52 Keyvan Kashkouli Nejad et al., "Spinal fMRI of Interoceptive Attention/ Awareness in Experts and Novices," *Neural Plasticity* 2014 (June 17, 2014): 679509, https://doi.org/10.1155/2014/679509.

53 Andrew Harver and Tyler S. Lorig, "Respiration," in *Handbook of Psychophysiology*, ed. J. T. Cacioppo, L. G. Tassinary, and G. G. Berntson (Cambridge, UK: Cambridge University Press, 2000); Peter D. Drummond et al., "Pain Increases during Sympathetic Arousal in Patients with Complex Regional Pain Syndrome," *Neurology* 57, no. 7 (2001): 1296–303, https://doi.org/10.1212/wnl.57.7.1296.

54 Deborah Badoud and Manos Tsakiris, "From the Body's Viscera to the Body's Image: Is There a Link between Interoception and Body Image Concerns?," *Neuroscience & Biobehavioral Reviews* 77 (2017): 237–46, https://doi.org/10.1016/j.neubiorev.2017.03.017; Cornelis J. E. Wientjes, "Respiration in Psychophysiology: Methods and Applications," *Biological Psychology* 34, no. 2–3 (1992): 179–203, https://doi.org/10.1016/0301-0511(92)90015-M; Mark E. Kunik et al., "Surprisingly High Prevalence of Anxiety and Depression in Chronic Breathing Disorders," *Chest* 127, no. 4 (2005): 1205–11, https://doi.org/10.1378/chest.127.4.1205.

55 William N. Gardner, "The Pathophysiology of Hyperventilation Disorders," *Chest* 109, no. 2 (1996): 516–34, https://doi.org/10.1378/chest.109.2.516; Lawrence M. Schleifer, Ronald Ley, and Thomas W. Spalding, "A Hyperventilation Theory of Job Stress and Musculoskeletal Disorders," *American Journal*

of Industrial Medicine 41, no. 5 (2002): 420–32, https://doi.org/10.1002/ajim.10061.

56 Christopher M. Worsham, Robert B. Banzett, and Richard M. Schwartzstein, "Air Hunger and Psychological Trauma in Ventilated Patients with COVID-19. An Urgent Problem," *Annals of the American Thoracic Society* 17, no. 8 (2020): 926, https://doi.org/10.1513/AnnalsATS.202004-322VP.

57 Jiangna N. Han et al., "Influence of Breathing Therapy on Complaints, Anxiety and Breathing Pattern in Patients with Hyperventilation Syndrome and Anxiety Disorders," *Journal of Psychosomatic Research* 41, no. 5 (1996): 481–93, https://doi.org/10.1016/S0022-3999(96)00220-6; Richard P. Brown and Patricia L. Gerbarg, "Sudarshan Kriya Yogic Breathing in the Treatment of Stress, Anxiety, and Depression: Part II—Clinical Applications and Guidelines," *Journal of Alternative and Complementary Medicine* 11, no. 4 (2005): 711–17, https://doi.org/10.1089/acm.2005.11.711; Volker Busch et al., "The Effect of Deep and Slow Breathing on Pain Perception, Autonomic Activity, and Mood Processing—An Experimental Study," *Pain Medicine* 13, no. 2 (2012): 215–28, https://doi.org/10.1111/j.1526-4637.2011.01243.x.

58 Ellen D. Hodnett and Richard W. Osborn, "Effects of Continuous Intrapartum Professional Support on Childbirth Outcomes," *Research in Nursing & Health* 12, no. 5 (1989): 289–97, https://doi.org/10.1002/nur.4770120504.

59 Mehling et al., "Body Awareness," 9.

Chapter 6

1 Melissa M. Karnaze and Linda J. Levine, "Lay Theories about whether Emotion Helps or Hinders: Assessment and Effects on Emotional Acceptance and Recovery from Distress," *Frontiers in Psychology* 11 (2020): 183, https://doi.org/10.3389/fpsyg.2020.00183.

2 Henriet van Middendorp et al., "Emotions and Emotional Approach and Avoidance Strategies in Fibromyalgia," *Journal of Psychosomatic Research* 64, no. 2 (2008): 159–67, https://doi.org/10.1016/j.psychores.2007.08.009, p. 165.

3 Anthony D. Ong et al., "Emodiversity and Biomarkers of Inflammation," *Emotion* 18, no. 1 (2018): 3–14, https://doi.org/10.1037/emo0000343.

4 Richard B. Lopez et al., "Emotion Regulation and Immune Functioning during Grief: Testing the Role of Expressive Suppression and Cognitive Reappraisal in Inflammation among Recently Bereaved Spouses," *Psychosomatic Medicine* 82, no. 1 (2020): 2–9, https://doi.org/10.1097/PSY.0000000000000755.

5 Jocelyn A. Sze et al., "Coherence between Emotional Experience and Physiology: Does Body Awareness Training Have an Impact?," *Emotion* 10, no. 6 (2010): 803–14, https://doi.org/10.1037/a0020146.

6 Jamil Zaki, Joshua Ian Davis, and Kevin N. Ochsner, "Overlapping Activity in Anterior Insula during Interoception and Emotional Experience," *NeuroImage* 62, no. 1 (2012): 493–99, https://doi.org/10.1016/j.neuroimage.2012.05.012.

7 Jurgen Fustos et al., "On the Embodiment of Emotion Regulation: Interoceptive Awareness Facilitates Reappraisal," *Social Cognitive and Affective Neuroscience* 8, no. 8 (2013): 911–17, https://doi.org/10.1093/scan/nns089.

8 Cynthia J. Price and Carole Hooven, "Interoceptive Awareness Skills for Emotion Regulation: Theory and Approach of Mindful Awareness in Body-Oriented Therapy (MABT)," *Frontiers in Psychology* 9 (2018): 798, https://doi.org/10.3389/fpsyg.2018.00798, p. 7.

9 Price and Hooven, 7.

10 Lisa R. Starr et al., "The Perils of Murky Emotions: Emotion Differentiation Moderates the Prospective Relationship between Naturalistic Stress Exposure and Adolescent Depression," *Emotion* 20, no. 6 (2020): 927–38, https://doi.org/10.1037/emo0000630.

11 Namiko Kamijo and Shintaro Yukawa, "The Role of Rumination and Negative Affect in Meaning Making Following Stressful Experiences in a Japanese Sample," *Frontiers in Psychology* 9 (2018): 2404, https://doi.org/10.3389/fpsyg.2018.02404.

12 Yuri Terasawa, Hirokata Fukushima, and Satoshi Umeda, "How Does Interoceptive Awareness Interact with the Subjective Experience of Emotion? An fMRI Study," *Human Brain Mapping* 34, no. 3 (2013): 598–612, https://doi.org/10.1002/hbm.21458.

13 John W. Burns, "Arousal of Negative Emotions and Symptom-Specific Reactivity in Chronic Low Back Pain Patients," *Emotion* 6, no. 2 (2006): 309–19, https://doi.org/10.1037/1528-3542.6.2.309.

14 Richard Stephens and Olly Robertson, "Swearing as a Response to Pain: Assessing Hypoalgesic Effects of Novel 'Swear' Words," *Frontiers in Psychology* 11 (2020): 723, https://doi.org/10.3389/fpsyg.2020.00723.

15 Evangelia Demerouti and Russell Cropanzano, "The Buffering Role of Sportsmanship on the Effects of Daily Negative Events," *European Journal of Work and Organizational Psychology* 26, no. 2, (2017): 263–74, https://doi.org/10.1080/1359432X.2016.1257610.

16 Frederic Nils and Bernard Rime, "Beyond the Myth of Venting: Social Sharing Modes Determine the Benefits of Emotional Disclosure," *European Journal of Social Psychology* 42, no. 6 (2012): 672–81, https://doi.org/10.1002/ejsp.1895.

17 David Gelles, "How to Be Mindful When You Are Angry," *New York Times*, April 5, 2017, https://nyti.ms/2oHtIve.

18 Yu Dong et al., "Managing Anxiety in the Medically Ill," *Psychiatric Times* 32, no. 1 (2015): 33, https://www.psychiatrictimes.com/view/managing-anxiety -medically-ill.

19 Murray B. Stein et al., "Increased Amygdala and Insula Activation during Emotion Processing in Anxiety-Prone Subjects," *American Journal of Psychiatry* 164, no. 2 (2007): 318–27, https://doi.org/10.1176/ajp.2007.164.2.318.

20 Barnaby D. Dunn et al., "Can You Feel the Beat? Interoceptive Awareness Is an Interactive Function of Anxiety- and Depression-Specific Symptom Dimensions," *Behaviour Research and Therapy* 48, no. 11 (2010): 1133–38, https://doi.org/10.1016/j.brat.2010.07.006; Sarah N. Garfinkel and Hugo D. Critchley, "Threat and the Body: How the Heart Supports Fear Processing," *Trends in Cognitive Sciences* 20, no. 1 (2016): 34–46, https://doi.org /10.1016/j.tics.2015.10.005; Jan Limmer, Johannes Kornhuber, and Alexandra Martin, "Panic and Comorbid Depression and Their Associations with Stress Reactivity, Interoceptive Awareness and Interoceptive Accuracy of Various Bioparameters," *Journal of Affective Disorders* 185, no. 1 (2015): 170–79, https://doi.org/10.1016/j.jad.2015.07.010.

21 Amelie J. A. A. Guyon et al., "Respiratory Variability, Sighing, Anxiety, and Breathing Symptoms in Low- and High-Anxious Music Students before and after Performing," *Frontiers in Psychology* 11 (2020): 303, https://doi.org /10.3389/fpsyg.2020.00303.

22 Jean Kim and Jack Gorman, "The Psychobiology of Anxiety," *Clinical Neuroscience Research* 4, no. 5–6 (2005): 335–47, https://doi.org/10.1016 /j.cnr.2005.03.008.

23 Mary Booker, "Working Creatively with Fear—An Inquiry," in *Cultural Landscapes in the Arts Therapies*, ed. Richard Hougham, Salvo Pitruzzella, and Sarah Scoble (Plymouth, UK: University of Plymouth Press, 2017), 151–72.

24 David Bercelli, *Trauma Releasing Exercises* (Self-Published, 2015).

25 Paul Ekman and Wallace V. Friesen, "Felt, False, and Miserable Smiles," *Journal of Nonverbal Behavior* 6, no. 4 (1982): 238–52, https://www.paulekman .com/wp-content/uploads/2013/07/Felt-False-And-Miserable-Smiles.pdf.

26 Paul Gilbert et al., "Feeling Safe and Content: A Specific Affect Regulation System? Relationship to Depression, Anxiety, Stress, and Self-Criticism," *Journal of Positive Psychology* 3, no. 3 (2008) 182–91, https://doi.org/10 .1080/17439760801999461.

27 Michelle N. Shiota et al., "Feeling Good: Autonomic Nervous System Responding in Five Positive Emotions," *Emotion* 11, no. 6 (2011): 1368–78, https://doi.org/10.1037/a0024278.

28 Corinna M. Perchtold-Stefan et al., "Motivational Factors in the Typical Display of Humor and Creative Potential: The Case of Malevolent Creativity," *Frontiers in Psychology* 11 (2020): 1213, https://doi.org/10.3389 /fpsyg.2020.01213.

29 Alan W. Gray, Brian Parkinson, and Robin I. Dunbar, "Laughter's Influence on the Intimacy of Self-Disclosure," *Human Nature* 26, no. 1 (2015): 28–43, https://doi.org/10.1007/s12110-015-9225-8.

30 Vanessa Pope, Rebecca Stewart, and Elaine Chew, "Audience Laughter Distribution in Live Stand-Up Comedy," in *Proceedings of Laughter Workshop*, ed. Jonathan Ginzburg and Catherine Pelachaud (Paris: Sorbonne University, 2018), 46–49.

31 Richard E. Boyatzis, Kyle Rochford, and Scott N. Taylor, "The Role of Positive Emotional Attractor in Vision and Shared Vision: Toward Effective Leadership, Relationships, and Engagement," *Frontiers in Psychology* 6 (2015): 670, https://doi.org/10.3389/fpsyg.2015.00670.

32 Bethany E. Kok et al., "How Positive Emotions Build Physical Health: Perceived Positive Social Connections Account for the Upward Spiral between Positive Emotions and Vagal Tone," *Psychological Science* 24, no. 7 (2013): 1123–32, https://doi.org/10.1177/0956797612470827.

33 Rollin McCraty and Maria A. Zayas, "Cardiac Coherence, Self-Regulation, Autonomic Stability, and Psychosocial Well-Being," *Frontiers in Psychology* 5 (2014): 1090, https://doi.org/10.3389/fpsyg.2014.01090.

34 David Huron and Jonna K. Vuoskoski, "On the Enjoyment of Sad Music: Pleasurable Compassion Theory and the Role of Trait Empathy," *Frontiers in Psychology* 11 (2020): 1060, https://doi.org/10.3389/fpsyg.2020.01060.

35 Helmuth Plessner, *Laughing and Crying: A Study of the Limits of Human Behavior* (Evanston, IL: Northwestern University Press, 2020), 132.

36 Plessner, 133–34.

37 Ad Vingerhoets and Jan Scheirs, "Sex Differences in Crying: Empirical Findings and Possible Explanations," in *Studies in Emotion and Social Interaction. Second Series. Gender and Emotion: Social Psychological Perspectives*, ed. A. H. Fischer (Cambridge, UK: Cambridge University Press, 2000), 143–65; James J. Gross, "Antecedent- and Response-Focused Emotion Regulation: Divergent Consequences for Experience, Expression, and Physiology," *Journal of Personality and Social Psychology* 74, no. 1 (1998): 224–37, https://doi.org/10.1037/0022-3514.74.1.224.

38 Lauren M. Bylsma et al., "When and for Whom Does Crying Improve Mood? A Daily Dairy Study of 1004 Crying Episodes," *Journal of Research in Personality* 45, no. 4 (2011): 385–92, https://doi.org/10.1016/j.jrp.2011.04.007.

39 Gwenda Simons et al., "Why Try (Not) to Cry: Intra- and Inter-Personal Motives for Crying Regulation," *Frontiers in Psychology* 3 (2013): 597, https://doi.org/10.3389/fpsyg.2012.00597.

40 Arnold B. Bakker and Ellen Heuven, "Emotional Dissonance, Burnout, and In-Role Performance among Nurses and Police Officers," *International Journal of Stress Management* 13, no. 4 (2006): 423–40, https://doi.org/10.1037/1072-5245.13.4.423.

41 Anne Gartner et al., "Emotion Regulation in Rescue Workers: Differential Relationship with Perceived Work-Related Stress and Stress-Related Symptoms," *Frontiers in Psychology* 9 (2019): 2744, https://doi.org/10.3389/fpsyg.2018.02744.

42 Kerstin Ryde, Maria Friedrichsen, and Peter Strang, "Crying: A Force to Balance Emotions among Cancer Patients in Palliative Home Care," *Palliative Support Care* 5, no. 1 (2007): 51–59, https://doi.org/10.1017/s1478951507070071.

43 Jonathan Rottenberg et al., "Vagal Rebound during Resolution of Tearful Crying among Depressed and Nondepressed Individuals," *Psychophysiology* 40, no. 1 (2003): 1–6, https://doi.org/10.1111/1469-8986.00001; James J. Gross, Barbara L. Fredrickson, and Robert W. Levenson, "The Psychophysiology of Crying," *Psychophysiology* 31, no. 5 (1994): 460–68, https://doi.org/10.1111/j.1469-8986.1994.tb01049.x.

44 Simons et al., "Why Try (Not) to Cry."

45 Ryde, Friedrichsen, and Strang, "Crying: A Force to Balance Emotions."

46 Amy J. C. Cuddy, Susan T. Fiske, and Peter Glick, "Warmth and Competence as Universal Dimensions of Social Perception: The Stereotype Content Model and the BIAS Map," in *Advances in Experimental Social Psychology: Vol. 40*, ed. M. P. Zanna (Cambridge, MA: Academic Press, 2008), 61–149.

47 Ad J. J. M. Vingerhoets, Niels Ven, and Yvonne Velden, "The Social Impact of Emotional Tears," *Motivation and Emotion* 40, no. 3 (2016): 455–63, https://doi.org/10.1007/s11031-016-9543-0.

48 Eileen Kennedy-Moore and Jeanne C. Watson, "How and When Does Emotional Expression Help?," *Review of General Psychology* 5, no. 3 (2001): 187–212, https://doi.org/10.1037/1089-2680.5.3.187.

49 Kennedy-Moore and Watson.

50 Susan Sussman, "The Significance of Psycho-Peristalsis and Tears within the Therapeutic Relationship," *Counselling and Psychotherapy Research* 1, no. 2 (2001): 90–100, https://doi.org/10.1080/14733140112331385128.

51 Chip Walter, "Why Do We Cry?," *Scientific American Mind* 17, no. 6 (2006): 44–51, https://doi.org/10.1038/scientificamericanmind1206-44.

52 C. Kingsley Mills and Arthur D. Wooster, "Crying in the Counselling Situation," *British Journal of Guidance and Counselling* 15, no. 2 (1987): 125–30, https://doi.org/10.1080/03069888700760161.

53 Judith Kay Nelson, *Seeing through Tears: Crying and Attachment* (Abingdon, UK: Taylor & Francis, 2005), 6.

54 Nelson, 217.

55 Leah S. Sharman et al., "Using Crying to Cope: Physiological Responses to Stress Following Tears of Sadness," *Emotion* 20, no. 7 (2020): 1279–91, https://doi.org/10.1037/emo0000633.

56 Dave Itzkoff, "The Lynn Sheldon That Marc Maron Knew," *New York Times*, July 31, 2020, https://nyti.ms/3hUNM8d.

57 Frank W. Wicker, Glen C. Payne, and Randall D. Morgan, "Participant Descriptions of Guilt and Shame," *Motivation and Emotion* 7, no. 1 (1983): 25–39, https://doi.org/10.1007/BF00992963; June Price Tangney and Ronda L. Dearing, *Shame and Guilt* (New York: Guilford, 2003).

58 Diana-Mirela Candea and Aurora Szentagotai-Tatar, "Shame-Proneness, Guilt-Proneness and Anxiety Symptoms: A Meta-analysis," *Journal of Anxiety Disorders* 58 (2018): 78–106, https://doi.org/10.1016/j.janxdis.2018.07.005.

59 Sarah G. Moore et al., "Coping with Condom Embarrassment," *Psychology, Health & Medicine* 11, no. 1 (2006): 70–79, https://doi.org/10.1080/13548500500093696.

60 Aaron D. Arndt and Ceren Ekebas-Turedi, "Do Men and Women Use Different Tactics to Cope with the Embarrassment of Buying Condoms?," *Journal of Consumer Behaviour* 16, no. 6 (2017): 499–510, https://doi.org/10.1002/cb.1648.

61 Heidi Fung, "Becoming a Moral Child: The Socialization of Shame among Young Chinese Children," *Ethos* 27, no. 2 (1999): 180–209, https://doi.org/10.1525/eth.1999.27.2.180.

62 Ken-Ichiro Okano, "Shame and Social Phobia: A Transcultural Viewpoint," *Bulletin of the Menninger Clinic* 58, no. 3 (1994): 323–38, https://psycnet.apa.org/record/1995-02040-001.

63 Sana Sheikh, "Cultural Variations in Shame's Responses: A Dynamic Perspective," *Personality and Social Psychology Review* 18, no. 4 (2014): 387–403, https://doi.org/10.1177/1088868314540810.

64 Matthew Feinberg, Robb Willer, and Dacher Keltner, "Flustered and Faithful: Embarrassment as a Signal of Prosociality," *Journal of Personality and Social Psychology* 102, no. 1 (2012): 81–97, https://doi.org/10.1037/a0025403.

65 Paula M. Niedenthal, "Embodying Emotion," *Science* 316, no. 5827 (2007): 1002–5, https://doi.org/10.1126/science.1136930; Mary Helen Immordino-Yang, "Me, My 'Self' and You: Neuropsychological Relations between Social Emotion, Self-Awareness, and Morality," *Emotion Review* 3, no. 3 (2011): 313–15, https://doi.org/10.1177/1754073911402391.

Chapter 7

1 Lawrence Kushner, *Honey from the Rock* (New York: Harper & Row, 1977), 22.

2 Louise Livingstone, "Dialoguing with Nature through the Thought of the Heart," in *In Other Tongues*, ed. Stuart Mugridge and Richard Povall (Totnes, UK: art.earth, 2018), 9.

3 Miriam-Rose Ungunmerr-Bauman, "Editorial. Against Racism," *Compass* 37, no. 3 (2003), http://compassreview.org/spring03/1.html.

4 Alycia Scott Zollinger, "The Art and Science of Somatic Praxis," *International Body Psychotherapy Journal* 19, 1 (Spring/Summer 2020): 64-74, https://ibpj.org/issues/IBPJ-Volume-19-Number-1-2020.pdf, p. 71.

5 Carol Burstein, "Living Inquiry," in *The Body in Psychotherapy: Inquiries in Somatic Psychology*, ed. Don Hanlon Johnson and Ian J. Grand (Berkeley, CA: North Atlantic Books, 1998), 118.

6 Danielle Elliot, "How a Virus Triage Tent Became a Serene Oasis for Health Care Workers." *New York Times*, June 12, 2020, https://www.nytimes.com/2020/06/12/nyregion/coronavirus-doctors-mental-health.html.

7 Marie I. Thouin-Savard, "Erotic Mindfulness: A Core Educational and Therapeutic Strategy in Somatic Sexology Practices," *International Journal of Transpersonal Studies* 38, no. 1 (2019), https://doi.org/10.24972/ijts.2019.38.1.203.

8 Nicole Daedone, *Slow Sex: The Art and Craft of the Female Orgasm* (New York: Grand Central Life & Style, 2011), 171.

9 Kimerer L. LaMothe, *Why We Dance: A Philosophy of Bodily Becoming* (New York: Columbia University Press, 2015).

10 Kimerer L. LaMothe, *What a Body Knows: Finding Wisdom in Desire* (United Kingdom: John Hunt Publishing, 2009), 146, 151–52.

11 Einat Shuper-Engelhard, "Ghosts in the Bedroom: Embodiment Wishes in Couple Sexuality: Qualitative Research and Practical Application," *American Journal of Dance Therapy* 41, no. 2 (2019): 302–17, https://doi.org/10.1007/s10465-019-09302-w.

12 David M. Lee et al., "Sexual Health and Positive Subjective Well-Being in Partnered Older Men and Women," *Journals of Gerontology Series B: Psychological Sciences and Social Sciences* 71, no. 4 (2016): 698–710, https://doi.org/10.1093/geronb/gbw018.

13 Bianca Fileborn et al., "Sex, Desire and Pleasure: Considering the Experiences of Older Australian Women," *Sexual and Relationship Therapy* 30, no. 1 (2015): 117–30, https://doi.org/10.1080/14681994.2014.936722, p. 121.

14 Fileborn et al., 122.

15 Fileborn et al., 122.

16 Fileborn et al., 123.

17 Annie Potts et al., "'Sex for Life'? Men's Counter-stories on 'Erectile Dysfunction,' Male Sexuality and Ageing," *Sociology of Health & Illness* 28, no. 3 (2006): 306–29, https://doi.org/10.1111/j.1467-9566.2006.00494.x, p. 317.

18 Potts et al., 320.

19 Jesse E. A. Verschuren et al., "Chronic Disease and Sexuality: A Generic Conceptual Framework," *Journal of Sex Research* 47, no. 2–3 (2010): 153–70, https://doi.org/10.1080/00224491003658227; Mitchell S. Tepper, "Letting Go of Restrictive Notions of Manhood: Male Sexuality, Disability and

Chronic Illness," *Sexuality and Disability* 17, no. 1 (1999): 37–52, https://doi.org/10.1023/A:1021451712988.

20 Alison M. Rhodes, "Claiming Peaceful Embodiment through Yoga in the Aftermath of Trauma," *Complementary Therapies in Clinical Practice* 21, no. 4 (2015): 247–56, http://dx.doi.org/10.1016/j.ctcp.2015.09.004, p. 251.

21 Laura Galbusera, Lisa Fellin, and Thomas Fuchs, "Towards the Recovery of a Sense of Self: An Interpretative Phenomenological Analysis of Patients' Experience of Body-Oriented Psychotherapy for Schizophrenia," *Psychotherapy Research* 29, no. 2 (2019): 234–50, https://doi.org/10.1080/10503307.2017.1321805, p. 6.

22 Barbara Holifield, "Against the Wall: Her Beating Heart," in *The Body in Psychotherapy: Inquiries in Somatic Psychology*, ed. Don Hanlon Johnson and Ian J. Grand (Berkeley, CA: North Atlantic Books, 1998), 63.

23 Sabine C. Koch and Beatrix Weidinger-von der Recke, "Traumatised Refugees: An Integrated Dance and Verbal Therapy Approach," *The Arts in Psychotherapy* 36, no. 5 (2009): 289–96, https://doi.org/10.1016/j.aip.2009.07.002, p. 292.

24 Amanda Lundvik Gyllensten et al., "Embodied Identity—A Deeper Understanding of Body Awareness," *Physiotherapy Theory and Practice* 26, no. 7 (2010): 439–46, https://doi.org/10.3109/09593980903422956, p. 443.

25 Tina Stromsted, "Embodied Imagination: Form Grows from Emptiness," in *Evocations of Absence: Interdisciplinary Encounters with Void States*, ed. Paul Ashton (New Orleans, LA: Spring Journal Books, 2007), 137–38.

26 Stromsted, 145.

27 Jon Julius Frederickson, Irene Messina, and Alessandro Grecucci, "Dysregulated Anxiety and Dysregulating Defenses: Toward an Emotion Regulation Informed Dynamic Psychotherapy," *Frontiers in Psychology* 9 (2018): 2054, https://doi.org/10.3389/fpsyg.2018.02054.

28 Mehling et al., "Body Awareness," 9.

29 Øystein Nødtvedt et al., "'You Feel They Have a Heart and Are Not Afraid to Show It': Exploring How Clients Experience the Therapeutic Relationship in Emotion-Focused Therapy," *Frontiers in Psychology* 10 (2019): 1996, https://doi.org/10.3389/fpsyg.2019.01996, p. 3.

30 Francine Lapides, "The Implicit Realm in Couples Therapy: Improving Right Hemisphere Affect-Regulating Capabilities," *Clinical Social Work Journal* 39, no. 2 (2011): 161–69, https://doi.org/10.1007/s10615-010-0278-1, p. 167.

31 Price and Hooven, "Interoceptive Awareness Skills," 9.

32 Cynthia Price et al., "Perceived Helpfulness and Unfolding Processes in Body-Oriented Therapy Practice," *Indo-Pacific Journal of Phenomenology* 11, no. 2 (2011): 1–15, https://doi.org/10.2989/IPJP.2011.11.2.5.1164, p. 11.

33 Price et al., 12.

34 Fanny Airosa et al., "Caring Touch as a Bodily Anchor for Patients after Sustaining a Motor Vehicle Accident with Minor or No Physical Injuries—A Mixed Methods Study," *BMC Complementary and Alternative Medicine* 16, no. 1 (2016): 106, https://doi.org/10.1186/s12906-016-1084-2, p. 5.

35 Fogel, "Practitioner Observations of Their Clients," 13–14.

36 Shantika Bernard, "Relational Somatic Presence—Meeting Trauma in Rosen Method Bodywork," *Rosen Method International Journal* 9, no. 1 (2016): 25–53, https://1xhdko41sric25njz22ditir-wpengine.netdna-ssl.com/wp-content/uploads/2016/09/BernardFinalArticleSpring2016.pdf, p. 41

37 Bernard, 43.

38 Susanna Jennifer Smart, "Grounded Theory of Rosen Method Bodywork" (PhD diss., Kent State University, Ohio, 2018), 130.

39 Smart, 133.

40 Smart, 157.

41 Antonie Lutz et al., "Investigating the Phenomenological Matrix of Mindfulness-Related Practices from a Neurocognitive Perspective," *American Psychologist* 70, no. 7 (2015): 632, https://doi.org/10.1037/a0039585.

42 Madhav Goyal et al., "Meditation Programs for Psychological Stress and Well-Being: A Systematic Review and Meta-analysis," *JAMA Internal Medicine* 174, no. 3 (2014) 357–68, https://doi.org/10.1001/jamainternmed.2013.13018; David R. Vago and David A. Silbersweig, "Self-Awareness, Self-Regulation, and Self-Transcendence (S-ART): A Framework for Understanding the Neurobiological Mechanisms of Mindfulness," *Frontiers in Human Neuroscience* 6 (2012): 296, https://doi.org/10.3389/fnhum.2012.00296; Britta K. Holzel et al., "Neural Mechanisms of Symptom Improvements in Generalized Anxiety Disorder Following Mindfulness Training," *NeuroImage: Clinical* 2 (2013): 448–58, https://doi.org/10.1016/j.nicl.2013.03.011; Yi-Yuan Tang, Britta K. Holzel, and Michael I. Posner, "The Neuroscience of Mindfulness Meditation," *Nature Reviews Neuroscience* 16 (2015): 213–25, https://doi.org/10.1038/nrn3916; Alberto Chiesa and Peter Malinowski, "Mindfulness-Based Approaches: Are They All the Same?," *Journal of Clinical Psychology* 67, no. 4 (2011): 404–24, https://doi.org/10.1002/jclp.20776.

43 David Treleaven, "Meditation, Trauma and Contemplative Dissociation," *Somatics* 16, no. 2 (2010): 20–22, http://ciis.academia.edu/DavidTreleaven/Papers/407288/Meditation_Trauma_and_Contemplative_Dissociation.

44 Anna Lutkajtis, "The Dark Side of Dharma: Why Have Adverse Effects of Meditation Been Ignored in Contemporary Western Secular Contexts?," *Journal for the Academic Study of Religion* 31, no. 2 (2018): 192–217, https://doi.org/10.1558/jasr.37053, p. 196.

45 Cimen Ekici, Gulcan Garip, and William Van Gordon, "The Lived Experiences of Experienced Vipassana Mahasi Meditators: An Interpretative Phenomenological

Analysis," *Mindfulness* 11, no. 1 (2020): 140–52, https://doi.org/10.1007/s12671-018-1063-4, p. 144.

46 Ekici, Garip, and Van Gordon, 146.

47 Ekici, Garip, and Van Gordon, 148.

48 Eric Van Lente and Michael J. Hogan, "Understanding the Nature of Oneness Experience in Meditators Using Collective Intelligence Methods," *Frontiers in Psychology* 11 (2020): 2092, https://doi.org/10.3389/fpsyg.2020.02092, p. 9.

49 Van Lente and Hogan, 10.

50 Van Lente and Hogan, 11.

51 Shepherd, *Radical Wholeness*, 167.

52 Steindl-Rast, *Way of Silence,* 46–47.

53 Terrell R. Moye and Joseph B. Westfall, "Spirituality & Medicine," *South Florida Hospital News and Healthcare Report* 5, no. 1 (December 2008), https://southfloridahospitalnews.com/page/Spirituality__Medicine/3613/1/.

54 Annick Shaw, Stephen Joseph, and P. Alex Linley, "Religion, Spirituality, and Posttraumatic Growth: A Systematic Review," *Mental Health, Religion & Culture* 8, no. 1 (2005): 1–11, https://doi.org/10.1080/1367467032000157981.

Index

About the Author

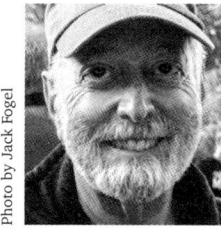

Photo by Jack Fogel

Alan Fogel, PhD, is a professor of psychology emeritus at the University of Utah and has been an active contributor to research on emotional development in human relationships from infancy through adulthood. His books include *Developing through Relationships* (1993, Chicago), *Infancy: Infant, Family, and Society*, 6th edition (2014, Sloan), and *Body Sense: The Science and Practice of Embodied Self-Awareness* (2013, Norton). Fogel is also a licensed massage therapist, a Rosen Method bodywork practitioner and senior teacher, and founding editor of the *Rosen Method International Journal*. He has a part-time practice in embodied self-awareness consulting and Rosen Method bodywork. Further information and links to publications can be found at http://www .alanfogelrosenmethod.abmp.com/ and at https://www.linkedin.com/in /alan-fogel-701a03122/. When not working, he finds restoration in gardening, singing and playing guitar, hiking and skiing in the mountains near his home in Salt Lake City, swimming and biking, and being with family and friends.

Γ Γ

ʒ/ /0

About North Atlantic Books

North Atlantic Books (NAB) is a 501(c)(3) nonprofit publisher committed to a bold exploration of the relationships between mind, body, spirit, culture, and nature. Founded in 1974, NAB aims to nurture a holistic view of the arts, sciences, humanities, and healing. To make a donation or to learn more about our books, authors, events, and newsletter, please visit www.northatlanticbooks.com.